# BE
# YOUTHFUL

# BE YOUTHFUL

Look Good, Feel Great—and
Remain Young at Any Age

Dr. Shino Bay Aguilera

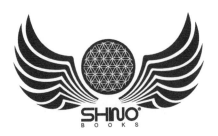

Miami, Florida

Copyeditor: Stephanie Gunning
Interior and cover design: Gus Yoo
Cover photo: Antonio Cuellar Photography

Shino Bay Books
350 Las Olas Boulevard, Suite 110
Fort Lauderdale, FL. 33301
www.beyouthfulbook.com
(954) 765-3005

978-0-9911445-0-1 (paperback)
978-0-9911445-1-8 (ebook)

1. Beauty 2. Health 3. Anti-aging 4. Personal grooming
5. Skin care 6. Dermatology 7. Cosmetics

*I dedicate this book to my beautiful grandmother,
Carmen, who taught me to be strong
in the midst of adversity and inspired me
to become a compassionate doctor.*

# Contents

# Preface

As a cosmetic dermatologist, I hear the same questions day after day during my consultations with patients:
"How can I avoid aging?"
"With all the sun damage I've got, do I have any hope?"
"What can I do to avoid getting a facelift?"

Everyone I meet appears to be desperately fighting to slow down the clock. Oftentimes, people arrive on the doorstep of my office with bagsful of lotions, potions, and serums, seeking my opinion on their beauty regimens. They want to know which of these ingredients hold the promise of being their perfect anti-aging solution. Many also come to me with their own preexisting ideas of how they would like me to use fillers, Botox®, and lasers to combat their ongoing processes of aging. These days, aging is a fight no one is willing to lose.

The battle I'm describing is partly the result of our obsession with youth in Western culture. But it's also because medicine has advanced swiftly in recent decades. We are living longer and we want our appearance to match. Not only do we want to have longevity; we want to feel great and look great, too. It is almost considered an insult to call someone old in our era.

Our current preoccupation with youth is not new; similar sentiments have been documented throughout history. The ancient quest to locate the healing waters of the legendary Fountain of Youth was pursued for more than a thousand years by notable explorers like Ponce de Leon, the European who discovered Puerto Rico and Florida. The quest for youth has been a constant, albeit largely unsuccessful pursuit—until lately. Recently, we've made real progress in this area.

Now, we have a viable youth restorer. Would you like to know what this new fountain of youth is that has been discovered? It's a combination of ways we can take care of ourselves so that we remain healthy on the inside and on the outside. Many factors contribute to our ability to maintain our youthfulness, including simple lifestyle modifications like a good skin care regimen.

During my consultations, while my patients are telling me their concerns about their appearance, I sit quietly and study their faces. I am trying to determine what's causing them to age. I am never concerned with their chronological age. Instead, I am concerned with their *apparent age*. There are both intrinsic and extrinsic factors that speed up the aging process. *Intrinsic factors* are issues related to internal health, such as diet, exercise, sleep, and stress. *Extrinsic factors* are environmental matters, such as sun exposure and pollution. Generally speaking, no single factor is ever the sole contributor to an aging face.

## HOW TO USE THIS BOOK

In *Be Youthful*, you'll learn what to do to keep your skin healthy and young looking during every decade of your life. I'm providing you with the same exact information and advice I give my own patients at Shino Bay Cosmetic Dermatology, Plastic Surgery & Laser Institute.

In Chapter 1, we discuss the importance of healthy fat to

maintaining a youthful appearance beyond midlife. In Chapter 2, the problem of how bone loss impacts appearance is explained. We look at the proportions and symmetry that make our faces appear aesthetically pleasing.

In Chapter 3, I describe the different layers of the skin and talk about the importance of collagen and elastic fibers. Here, I also go into detail about intrinsic and extrinsic factors that age the skin. Smoking and sunlight are primary culprits.

Chapter 4 is devoted to the most common maladies of the skin: acne, rosacea, eczema, wrinkles, scars, melasma, and blemishes. Mostly benign conditions, I nonetheless call these the "seven plagues."

In Chapter 5, we take a deep dive into the subject of sun damage and photoaging, which is responsible for most of the wrinkles and brown spots we see as we get older. You'll learn about different wavelengths of ultraviolet light and how to safeguard your youthful skin from all of them. There is much confusion about sun protection. Here you'll gain clarity.

In Chapter 6, you'll be brought decade by decade from your twenties to your sixties and beyond to discover the physical changes the body goes through and how these are likely to impact your skin and alter your appearance as you age. I make specific recommendations for which kinds of moisturizers, cleansers, and treatments are appropriate and necessary for people at different ages to use. There's a special section for women on preparing for menopause.

In Chapter 7, we explore the world of neuromodulators: Botox, Dysport, and Xeomin. Similarly, in Chapter 8, we explore the subject of injectable dermal fillers—silicone, fat transfers, collagen, and hyaluronic acids among them—as well as autologous plasma and stem cell injections. The term *autologous* simply means that these are done with an individual's own plasma and stem cells, which have been medically prepared for this specific purpose.

In Chapter 9, I go into great detail about my favorite device:

the laser. Lasers of different wavelengths can be used to treat different skin tones and issues that present in tones that span the range of the color palette. Here, I describe the best devices on the market today for treating unwanted hair, vascular lesions, wrinkles, photoaging, and more.

Lotion and potions are covered in Chapter 10. What's the difference between retinoids and hydroxy acids? When should you take DMAE or vitamins?  What about peptides? Here's where we explore antioxidants, botanicals, and cosmeceuticals—even snail slime!

In Chapter 11, we take a look at how feeling beautiful or handsome comes from within as much as from without.

Chapter 12 is a wonderful chapter contributed by my dear friend Loren Psaltis, who has worked in many capacities in the beauty industry throughout her career, including working as an elite makeup artist. Loren is an accomplished woman. Among other things she's done, she developed an in-house brand of cosmetics for a department store chain and served as a marketing director for Calvin Klein. As is done in Chapter 6, the material in Chapter 12 is organized according to decade beginning in your twenties and continuing to your sixties and beyond. Loren first describes the tools of the makeup trade, such as brushes, tweezers, sponges, and eyelash curlers. Then she explains primers, foundation, concealers, and powders; blushes and contouring; and corrective techniques for different eye shapes.

In Chapter 13, we explore how attitude contributes to vitality and youthfulness. If we live as if we're young, we feel younger than if we surrender to the clock. Exercise, nutrition, the force of gravity, and good mental health are all important to keeping us youthful, active, curious, participating, and happy.

## REMEMBER, BEAUTY IS AGELESS

The best antiaging advice I could give you is to look within. Since external beauty fades and youth comes with an expiration date, if we want to be perceived as beautiful or handsome for a lifetime we must find our inner beauty. As a cosmetic dermatologist, I deal with people's vanity, fears, and nightmares. Although it is my karma and God-given talent as a medical doctor to help my patients reverse or defy the aging processes and stay young looking, my work goes beyond simple appearances.

Within my heart I understand that I am here to give the individuals under my care spiritual facelifts, and help them awaken the life force within them that will allow them to achieve their goals. Once this life force is activated in you, you'll understand that your beauty is ageless. Youth is a state of mind. Love and kindness are the real elixirs of eternal youth.

Above everything else, make a point of being kind to yourself. You can reduce stress by practicing self-acceptance and staying positive. Let go of resentments and build relationships where you give and receive love, affection, and encouragement. Staying young is about having the willingness to try new things and being curious about life. Apply the wisdom that comes with experience and advancing years to accepting yourself and loving body, mind, and spirit.

Shino Bay Aguilera, D.O.
Fort Lauderdale, Florida
June 2014

# CHAPTER 1

# Fat Is Your Friend

Some of the information I share with my patients surprises them. After listening to their concerns for a while, I may, for instance, ask, "Did you know that *fat* is one of the key ingredients in the fountain of youth you're seeking?"

At this point, they typically look back at me incredulously. Their eyes open wide, and then there is a chuckle. Finally they come to the realization that I am being serious.

When my patients ask me my age, I reply that I am in my forties. Because I look about half that age, knowing my age helps them start to believe that maybe I do have some answers on how to slow down or reverse aging. Some people get confused when they see my super-thin frame, which has hardly an ounce of fat on it. "But you are very thin," they point out. "How can fat possibly be the fountain of youth?"

I reply, "The fountain of youth is not the fat on your body. It's the fat in your face!"

## THE FAT STORY

The world has become downright fat phobic. This is due, in part, to scientific evidence that obesity (excessive stored body fat, especially in the area of the belly) may be responsible for diseases ranging from heart disease to diabetes and some forms of cancer. In response, some people have declared a fight against fat and refuse to consume it. Many people believe that the fats in our food turn into fat on our bodies. With so many people in this country struggling with being overweight and the corresponding health issues, it is no surprise that many feel an animosity toward dietary fats, which they were taught in the past were their enemy. But this is a misconception. Obesity doesn't result exclusively from overconsumption of a single nutrient.

Fortunately, in recent years we have learned that not all fats are unhealthy to eat. In fact, there are even "good fats," such as those found in salmon and other oily fish, walnuts, flaxseeds, avocadoes, and olive oil. Good fats aid in metabolic processes, help fight off diseases, and are essential for the health of the human body. Fats help improve the functions of different organs and systems of the body, including:

- **The brain:** Fats make up 60 percent of the brain and are essential to several brain functions, including learning, memory, and mood. Fats are especially important for women to eat during pregnancy, as they are essential for the development of the fetal brain.
- **The cells:** Fatty acids on the cells' surfaces help them to stay flexible and are responsible for building cellular membranes.
- **The nerves:** The material that insulates and protects the nerves is composed of fat. Fat aids in isolating their electrical impulses and speeding up the transmission of signals from parts of the body to the brain.
- **The eyes:** Fat cushions and protects the eyes, and it is essential for their optimal functioning.

- **The heart:** Specific fats are essential to help the heart beat in a regular rhythm. Sixty percent of the heart's energy comes directly from burning fat.
- **The lungs:** Saturated fats are essential for the production of the lung surfactants that keep the lungs from collapsing. These fats come from sources such as chicken, red meat, dairy, coconut oil, and palm oil.
- **The digestive system:** Fat slows the digestive process so that the body has more time to absorb required nutrients. Also, vitamins A, D, E, and K actually require fat for absorption.
- **The immune system:** Inflammation, which plays a huge role in aging, is attenuated by fat, which helps the immune system and the metabolism to function properly.
- **All internal organs:** Omental fat (the kind that is stored within the tissue that supplies your intestines with blood) protects and cushions all internal organs.

As you can see, fats play an integral role in the well-being of the human body. They protect internal organs by providing energy, fueling building blocks for hormones, and by absorbing fat-soluble vitamins. That being said, an accumulation of fat in the body generally reflects an unhealthy lifestyle (inactivity and/or overeating) or a genetic predisposition to put on padding. Unhealthy weight, especially fat stored in the belly, is considered a harbinger of potential medical problems and is not aesthetically pleasing.

Interestingly, however, facial fat is one of most important tissues that affect the aging face. In recent studies, the medical community has found that deep subcutaneous facial fat gives the face its youthful position, contour, and dimensions. Facial fat is critical in slowing down the morphological changes that occur to our faces over time. When we lose too much facial fat, we begin to look gaunt and aged.

You can appreciate the value of fat in a person's face when you see people who have lost a lot of weight. Their bodies may look amazing, but their faces look as if they have aged significantly. For all these years, most of us have been trying to keep our body fat percentage at a minimum without knowing that our faces were being negatively affected. Indeed, it is ironic that much-hated fat is actually what maintains our youthful features and keeps us from running to a plastic surgeon.

Unfortunately, each of us has an internal clock on our facial fat cells that determines how soon they will start disappearing and thereby cause the volume depletion of our faces. Some of us, due to genetic factors, will lose our facial fat cells slower than others. This is why some people, even those with sun-damaged skin, can appear younger than their peers of the same age; and why those who "do everything right" age drastically fast.

Another factor that affects facial fat cells is the pressure we put on our faces when we are sleeping. If we favor one side of the face while sleeping, that side of the face will always appear older than the other. This is because the side of the face that is pressed down on the pillow or arm is not getting the same amount of oxygen and nutrients as the other side. The fat cells of the affected area become starved, then begin to deflate and eventually vanish. This is how I can tell which side of the bed a patient sleeps on. The affected side appears pushed back and droops while the unaffected side tends to look plump and younger.

During consultations, I usually lift up a mirror to demonstrate how one side of the face looks younger, while the other side has deeper nasolabial folds (lines from the corner of the nose to the corner of the mouth) and fleshier jowls. Patients tend to be unaware of the different rates of aging because they are usually only focusing on the secondary effects of losing fat volume on their faces. Since symmetry equates to beauty, if you have an asymmetrical face it is robbing you of your natural beauty and attractiveness.

## THE TRIANGLE OF YOUTH VS. THE PYRAMID OF OLD AGE

The face can be divided into thirds: an upper third, a middle third, and a lower third. During our youth, there is a smooth transition of the tissues from one area to the next. As we age, we begin to lose the strategically placed facial fat that serves as a scaffold for the structures above it. The skin also begins to show a loss of elasticity and a decrease in thickness, rendering it unable to accommodate the volume loss in the underlying tissues. The smooth transitions we once enjoyed become bumpier. This is the beginning of the aging process. We look aged when we no longer have the same facial contour that we had in our twenties and thirties. Of course, this is just the softer appearance of being middle aged. An elderly face comes later with bone loss.

In our youth, the widest part of the face is the area beneath the cheekbones that narrows down to the chin like an inverted triangle. This area is known as the *triangle of youth* (see figure 1a below). With age, the forehead narrows due to temporal atrophy; it also elongates, causing the brow line to drop. The lower face widens due to volume loss in the flesh over the cheekbones, leading to sagging and jowling. The jawbone also gets remodeled and parts of its mass are reabsorbed. All of these changes causes the triangle of youth to become the *pyramid of old age* (see figure 1b below).

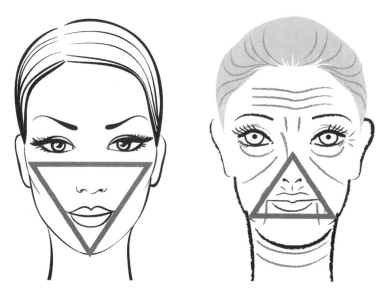

**Figures 1a and 1b.** The triangle of youth **(figure 1a)** is delineated by the cheekbones and chin. The pyramid of old age **(figure 1b)** is delineated by the two sides of the jawbone below our ears and the center of the forehead.

Every structure in the human body is interconnected. Changes in individual tissues are interrelated; alterations in one type of tissue (for example, fat, bone, skin, or muscle) lead to modifications in the other types of tissue. The whole collection of changes is what causes a change in an individual's overall facial appearance as he or she ages. For example, volume loss of the deep midfacial fat results in decreased support of the medial cheek compartment. This results in a diminished midface projection (in other words, a flattening of the face) and the unmasking of nasolabial folds. This occurs because the malar fat, or mid-cheek fat, seems to slide forward and down with age. These phenomena, combined with gravity, create a negative vector—a downward force—in which excessive traction is placed on the skin of the lower eyelid, causing it to lengthen and lose elasticity.

Because of the way fat is originally located in our faces, in youth we are given the well-rounded, three-dimensional topography that we desperately seek to maintain as we get older.

This subcutaneous facial fat is partitioned into discrete compartments that age independently from one another. For this reason, it is possible to see a decrease in the volume of facial fat in some areas and an accumulation of fat volume in others. As time goes by, transitions from one part of the face to the others get disrupted, creating shadows and malpositioning of the defining arcs of a youthful face. The fullness and roundness of the face gets broken up into uneven planes, creating a more drawn and aged appearance.

Ultimately, bone loss due to reabsorption leads to the pyramid of old age, in which there is a sagging downward descent of facial soft tissues that drape around the mouth.

## THE OLD "OLD FACE" METHOD

It was long theorized that facial aging was due to the relaxation of facial muscles. Therefore many surgical techniques and devices were created to tighten or shorten the facial muscles in order to rejuvenate the face. Different books and videos were sold that suggested electrical currents could be used to tone facial muscles. However, this theory had a critical flaw evidenced by observing patients with facial paralysis. The folds around the mouths, eyes, and between the eyebrows of those with facial nerve paralysis tend to soften and appear younger on the affected side. In addition, Botox® improves the appearance of wrinkles and creases by relaxing—not tightening—muscles around the eyes, between the forehead, and on the neck.

As a child, I remember my mother and grandmother doing all kinds of facial exercises—none of which seemed to help stop the aging of their faces. The Internet is full of sites claiming that isometric facial exercises that stimulate muscle tone prevent facial wrinkles. However, a study published in the *Journal of Aesthetic Plastic Surgery* by Le Louarn and colleagues (2007) suggests that repeated muscle contraction of the facial muscles actually can expel fats from deep compartments below the muscles into other compartments overlaying the muscles, causing malposition of facial fat, straightening and shortening of facial muscles, and overall decreased muscle tone. They also conducted MRI studies that examined the association of facial fat and muscles in people of various ages. This showed that the position of the fat determines the shape and subsequent action of the muscle. In addition, the MRI data also revealed that facial muscles have a curvilinear convex contour because of the underlying facial fat.

The authors of this study theorize that the acquired shape of the facial muscles, due to the underlying fat, dictates both the direction and amplitude of muscle contractions that are characteristic of a youthful facial expression. As we age, these muscles gradually straighten, shorten, and become more flaccid due to the volume depletion of the underlying fat. This is consistent with the earlier statement that changes in an individual tissue will lead to changes in other types of tissues, affecting an individual's overall appearance as he or she ages.

Other studies using MRI scans have found no difference in overall facial muscle thickness, length, or volume in patients over fifty-nine years in age and those between sixteen and thirty. Additionally, we know that using Botox to prevent the movement of facial muscles proves to be far more effective in preventing aging than the daily routine of exercising these muscles. It is the movement of these muscles during everyday living that contributes to the formation of the lines in the first place. The constant rubbing, pulling, and dragging of the skin in daily life causes mild inflammation. This, in turn, affects the integrity of the existing collagen and elastic fibers in the dermis, resulting in a less elastic, thinner, and dryer skin as time passes.

The use of muscle-toning systems tends to come in and out of style every so often. I can remember purchasing a device endorsed by actress Linda Evans that looked like a scary mask. It had a few metal contact plates that caused an electrical current to stimulate the facial muscles in a rhythmic pattern. I was able to control the intensity of the current and the pain threshold levels. Although I used it religiously for a few weeks, I never saw the improvements that were promised. The erroneous premise was that the aging process causes muscles to sag and lose their tone, leading to a dull, aged, and inelastic skin, so toning the muscles underneath the skin would reverse the process and lead to smoother, younger-looking skin. But there is little evidence that this approach to antiaging is effective.

Continuing my research, I also came across facial weights for muscle toning and development. The premise for the invention I tried was that by using steel-bead weights on the face and following up with a resistance exercise routine, the facial muscles could be toned and developed. Although there have been reports of facial weights helping people recover from facial paralysis and facial trauma, infection, and surgery, there is no data to support the notion that facial weight-resistance exercises improve the appearance or prevent the look of aging.

From the bizarre to the ridiculous, I have found devices that promise a non-surgical "facelift" via electric current stimulation. Their manufacturers all swear that the loss of muscle tonicity and mass are one of the major causes, if not the major cause, of aging and the sagging of facial skin. Old "Old Face" methods of treatment were all about muscle tone and mass, but New "Old Face" methods are about preventing volume loss of bones and facial fat compartments.

## THE NEW "OLD FACE" METHOD

For years it was believed that the human face could be restored to a more youthful state by subtractive methods, such as the removal of fat and skin. The surgery consisted of removing excess sagging skin and fat pads, and then pulling the tissues tightly. The aim was facial tightening. Unfortunately, this approach made older people look like they'd been through a wind tunnel, and announced to the world, "I have had a facelift." They did not look any younger after their facelifts; they just looked like old people who'd had work done on them. Pulling the skin and underlying tissues tightly over a volume-less face only leads to a cadaveric appearance.

Today's school of thought about facial rejuvenation is a paradigm shift. The emphasis has departed from the older, subtractive techniques to focus more on restorative methods. The latest techniques are designed to restore facial fat volume and contour the tissues in an attempt to emulate a younger and more natural looking face. The New "Old Face" method is all about fat and volume!

A young face has an ample amount of volume. This can easily be seen in the plump faces of babies. As we get older, however, fat is redistributed in strategic compartments to hold the face up. These fat compartments are independent from one another, meaning that not all will age at the same rate. However, they are also interdependent. Changes in one compartment will lead to changes in other fat compartments, as well as changes in other types of tissues.

Facial fat loss is highly individualized. Several factors determine how soon the fat on our faces vanishes. I have noticed that patients who have better volume in their faces always appear younger looking, even without having had any procedures.

But lifestyle can damage fat stores. Marathon runners and triathletes, who are constantly exerting themselves physically, have very little body fat. People who favor one side or lying face down on the mattress while sleeping can deplete the fat cells in one area. People who are wheelchair-bound or bedridden, for example, often have problems with bedsores. When very little oxygen or nutrients is flowing to a tissue, it causes that tissue to starve and begin to disappear. Although most of us do not spend enough hours lying on our faces at night to get bedsores, it still makes a difference. I call the appearance of having slept on one's face the "thumb-print sign" because the nice apples of the face in time become so flat and gaunt that it almost looks like someone has used his or her thumbs to push them in—like you would with clay.

For years, I have been educating my patients about the theory that fat keeps our appearance youthful. It is not hard to get them to agree with me because it's pure physics and biology 101. While there are other factors that affect the aging of our faces, none has the power to slow down the clock like facial fat and bone. Look at a picture of your grandparents when they were younger and to compare it to how they look now or right before they passed away. Obviously, there were pronounced changes in the morphology of their faces between the first and the second photos.

We can look at people and categorize them at a glance as either "young" or "old." When my grandmother was young, she was one of the most beautiful women you would ever see. Before she died, however, she began to look a little "witchy." If it were not for her beautiful hazel green eyes you could hardly have told that it was the same person. How did she change so drastically? The answer is that as her facial fat began to disappear and was redistributed according to the law of gravity. Bone resorption also took place. Volume loss and redistribution of fat are signs that other changes in the face, such as bone resorption, muscle lengthening, and skin flaccidity, are soon to follow.

Women need to be more vigilant than men about such changes due to the effects of menopause on the bones, collagen fibers, and elastic fibers of the skin. Fat loss starts taking place in women around the thirties, which is why I make a point to educate women of this age that come to see me for treatment about preparing ahead of time for the impact of menopause. No matter their age, but especially when they have the advantage of their youth, women need to do weight-bearing exercises and eat a balanced diet that will help them to increase their bone density and maintain an ideal body weight. They also need to avoid smoking, excessive sun exposure, and if possible, sleeping on their faces. In other words, they need to be vigilant in avoiding a deficit of any body tissues before they get to menopause.

Men also go through morphological facial changes as they age due to not having enough facial fat, though not at the same rate as women. It cannot hurt us to be diligent in our self-care either.

The deep fat compartments under the midfacial muscles are what give them their curvilinear round contours. At the widest part, they form what we call the apples of our faces. Over time, these fat stores start to taper off. With the help of gravity, the muscles start to lose their shape, and the face elongates and deflates like a balloon. The nice apples of the cheek then look more like saggy pancakes. Fat loss leaves the face looking flat or hollow and accentuates the lines known as nasolabial folds, which run from the sides of the nose to the corners of the mouth.

When I see patients who are mainly bothered by their deep nasolabial folds, I always take a close look at their cheeks. If I see that their folds are due to having faces that are deflating and dropping, I will not try to correct folds using fillers. Instead, I educate them using a little bit of physics. Imagine that your face is coming down and I add more weight to it. I would be helping gravity to create a downward vector that would accelerate the aging process. I see many patients that had done just that. After my explanations, they understand why they still do not look rested or younger after filling their lines. I will only fill these lines if they have a good midfacial volume. Otherwise, I correct the volume loss, and the nasolabial folds disappear right before their eyes without using any filler.

When we start to lose our mid-facial fat, we create a vertical downward negative vector that leads to excessive traction on the lower eyelid. This eventually leads to sclera show, a condition in which your lower lid drops and reveals more of the white part of the eye. This phenomenon is known as V-shaped deformity of the lower eyelid. Studies show that as we age there is a loss of elasticity of the fragile skin around our eyes. It's like having an old sock that has lost its elasticity from constant pulling and keeps slipping down around one's ankles. In order to prove this theory, scientists conducted a study that concluded that when medial cheek elevation was restored with fillers there was an improvement in the rapid return of the lower eyelid skin after being pinched. Pinching flesh in this manner is called a snap test.

I observe this phenomenon every day in my practice. When you improve the volume of a sunken cheek with filler you also improve the skin elasticity in the eye area and the skin around the mouth, jawline, and upper neck. This again evidences that our facial tissues are interdependent; changes in one affect the others.

Other strategic areas of importance for fat and tissue loss, especially for women, are the temples. These are often neglected or ignored, but they play an important role in preventing facial aging. As we age, the temples become increasingly hollow, making the forehead appear narrower—one of the signs of the pyramid of old age. This creates a negative vector that causes the upper eyelid to drop. This is also the reason why our eyes seem to get smaller and smaller as we age. When this ignored area of the face is finally addressed, it has a big impact in the rejuvenation of the face.

Several processes contribute to jowl formation. Ironically, it has to do with not enough and with too much facial fat all simultaneously. Have you ever heard the term skinny-fat? I have always felt that way. I am extremely thin, yet I can accumulate excess fat around my waist if I don't watch it. The same notion applies to the face. The face loses fat in certain areas, but it can accumulate some in others.

A similar process occurs with jowl formation. When the buccal fat around our mouth dimples starts to diminish in conjunction with the preauricular fat (the fat on the edges of the face right in front of the ears), it creates a forward movement of the face. Adding the downward and forward vectors of temporal wasting, the superficial fat accumulation along the jawline causes the chin to become the widest part of the face. In addition to all of these soft tissue changes, we also see bone loss and a repositioning of the chin and the jawline. A deficit in skeletal thickness and bone density further distorts the ratio of a youthful face.

The malar fat pad (the small area of fat that sits right above the cheekbone and under the lower eyelid like a small pillow), slides forward and downward and bulges against the nasolabial crease as we age. This, in turn, causes the under eye area to protrude due to fat pouch accumulation in this region.

It is not a secret that our eyes are floating around in fat. The eyes sit inside a bony socket that encloses a space known as the orbit. The border of this bony socket is called the orbital rim. In addition to the eyeball, the orbit contains an array of tiny muscles, blood vessels, and nerves that allow for the proper functioning of the eyes. Surrounding these structures sits the orbital fat, which is a sort of padding that protects and cushions all these delicate structures. Any process that depletes or disturbs the orbital fat is bound to have negative consequences in the appearance of the eye area. You can see, for example, that extremely malnourished people with little fat mass in their bodies tend to have a sunken and gaunt appearance around their eyes.

The ocular fat compartment is not immune to the loss of soft tissue fullness that comes with aging. As the orbital fat compartments begin to vanish, a person starts to appear tired and older. Later, the eyes become hollow and cast shadows, making the skin appear darker and indented. Finally, the atrophy of this fat compartment is so severe that sometimes you can actually see the orbital rim itself, giving a skeletal appearance to the face.

In the past, plastic surgeons often removed orbital fat during surgery (also known as blepharoplasty). This left their patients worse off than before. Unfortunately, this subtractive technique left many patients with very hollow looking eyes. At present, most plastic surgeons practice tissue-sparing techniques. Bulging fat is usually carefully returned to its normal anatomic compartment, making fat removal unnecessary. Excess fat removal and repositioning is now left for those patients who tend to suffer from extreme fat herniation under their eyes.

Facial fat is the master tissue that holds the secrets of a youthful face. Each one of us will lose facial fat according to our genetics, gender, and lifestyle. In addition, fat loss is highly individualized among compartments in the face. Each compartment will lose volume independently of the others, potentially leading to asymmetry of the face. This also causes the outer envelope of the face to fold or sag, regardless of how well someone might have taken care of his or her skin. This illustrates how changes in facial fat may influence changes in other tissues such as skin and muscle, and possibly bone. The New "Old Face" method is all about the appreciation of the importance of facial fat.

Although our culture has become increasingly fat phobic, we are now preaching the importance of fat as the most powerful weapon to slow down the clock. The awareness of the importance of facial fat may aid young women and men who suffer from eating disorders, including teenagers, to understand that a certain amount of fat in the body is healthy and necessary to maintain youth and vitality. As a former male model who earned a living doing underwear catalogs, I became obsessed with my weight. I tried to keep my body fat extremely low even though I was already thirty pounds underweight.

At six feet tall and weighing 135 pounds, I was unhealthfully thin. My abs, however, photographed great! Losing my abs represented losing my income. I was surrounded by young men and women who would do anything to be skinny for the same reasons as me. When you are young and obsessed with fat, it can easily lead to an unhealthy way of living that creates a recipe for disaster. Once you enter into this world, however, it can be difficult to get out. The more emotions that you attach to it, the lower you slide down the emotional grading scale. For those who hit rock bottom, it can sometimes even lead to fatal results. I hope that by creating a healthy awareness of the importance of fat in the aging process, I may help in my own small way to eliminate eating disorders. After all, most people would rather be a little overweight than look old.

# CHAPTER 2

# The "Darn Clock"!

Tick tock. There goes one second of our lives . . . a second we'll never get back.

Before the invention of the clock, time was a rather ambiguous and undefined concept that did not play an important role in people's lives. Most ancient civilizations measured time by the position of the sun. People worked as long as the sun was up and returned home to their families as the sun went down. The Egyptians measured time with sundials, and the Chinese used water clocks. During the middle ages, time was either measured by candles that burned in hourly increments or with hourglasses. As "time" went on and the ticking clock became a pervasive element in everyday life, managing time became a more important aspect of the human experience.

Scientists postulate that time is a physical force that plays an integral role in the happenings of the universe and in the human body. It is no longer just a way to reference the passage of events. Time is a force, a law that governs our internal and external experience. The relationship between time and self is intimately connected. The search for ways to beat the clock by having more time to accomplish the things we want to has therefore become an important pursuit. However, with the increase in life expectancy due to medical and technological advances, we realize that a greater quantity of time, in and of itself, is not sufficient unless we also feel and look good. For that reason, the *quality* of time has become the new object of our affection.

The concept of eternal *youth* (as distinct from eternal life) was well understood and illustrated in Greek and Roman mythology. In Western antiquity, however, living forever—while continuing to age—was considered a punishment rather than a blessing. Finding a way to stop or reverse the aging process has therefore become a relentless obsession for many people. The Spanish adventurer, Juan Ponce de Leon, believed in a legendary Fountain of Youth that would restore the vitality and appearance of anyone who drank from its waters. The quest for age reversal or agelessness was his holy grail.

During consultations, most of my patients report that although they still feel young and vital on the inside, how well they feel does not match their external appearances. It is not easy to bear witness to the morphological changes of your face and body when you still feel young and vivacious. However, it seems like every cell in our body has its own consciousness—and each has become aware of the biological "clock," too!

Who can forget Marisa Tomei's Oscar winning line in *My Cousin Vinnie*, "My biological clock is ticking like this—[*stomp, stomp, stomp*]!" It seems like everything in the human experience follows a clock. The ovaries follow it. Men's hair follicles follow it. As we've already discussed, our facial fat cells follow an internal clock. Recently, scientists discovered that the bony elements of the face also change significantly with age. There is ample data in medical literature that demonstrates a significant loss of volume in the craniofacial skeleton around age fifty for both men and women.

With patients who are seeking to slow down their aging process, I explain that the preservation of facial fat is a key component of the dermatological fountain of youth. But fat loss alone does not make anyone appear elderly; it simply makes us look older, gaunt, rough, or tired. We begin to acquire an elderly face when we start to experience bone loss on our cheeks and around the orbital rim of our eyes. When these bone changes occur, we have acquired the skull of an elderly person. Since fat loss tends to occur much sooner than bone loss, I urge my patients to tackle the problem of fat loss as soon as they notice any signs of it.

I usually use the analogy of a child with Down syndrome to describe how we determine if a person has an elderly face. No one has to tell us if a child has Down syndrome. It takes a quick glance and we know, because regardless of the race of the child, a child with Down syndrome has acquired a particular arrangement of skull bones that gives him or her a similar face or look. The same is true of an elderly person. Once the changes around the cheekbones and eyes occur, with one glance we can discern if a person is young or elderly. The bones of the skull are the platform of the face, and they dictate the shape and position of the fat, muscle, and skin tissues above them.

Imagine that the bony elements of the face act like a sturdy table, while the soft tissues of the face act like a tablecloth. As the table starts to shrink due to volume loss, it leaves less surface area to accommodate the tablecloth, causing it to fold or sag when it hits the floor. Shrinkage in craniofacial bone volume is more pronounced in women due to the effects of . . . *stomp, stomp, stomp* . . . menopause.

I often refer to the chin, also known as the lower jawbone, or *mandible,* as the floor of the face. The upper jawbone, or *maxilla,* articulates with the mandible to create fundamental movements that aid us in eating and speaking. The massive amounts of articulation and movement going on in this area create a multitude of expression lines as we age. The aging of the maxilla and the mandible contributes greatly to midfacial soft tissue descent. For this reason, the early signs of aging are always more pronounced around the mouth.

Using computed tomography (CT) scans and other imaging technology, scientists have discovered that with age there is a retrograde rotation of the maxilla, causing the teeth to be displaced to behind their earlier position. As we age, the mandible also begins to rotate downward and posterior due to bone resorption. In addition, the lack of skeletal height, or volume, in the maxilla causes the upper lip to slide down and roll inside the mouth, causing the top lip to appear thinner as we age. The shift of skeletal proportions in the mandible due to bone loss leads to malpositioning of the soft tissue in an accordion-like manner that dermatologists and plastic surgeons refer to as the concertina effect.

The concertina effect, simply put, is when the "tablecloth" of skin tissue hits the floor and starts to fold and sag. I have noticed that these changes are more pronounced and occur much earlier in life in patients who suffer from temporomandibular joint disorder (TMJ) or clench their teeth at night, or in those who have had a lot of dental work. The amount of mobility and articulation on the upper and lower jawbones causes the wear and tear on the bones and loss of bone mass. Whenever I see a forty-something woman with changes around her mouth that are usually attributed to bone loss, I may ask her if she has any of these issues. She is usually astonished about my guess.

"Well, I am not a psychic," I say. When I see changes around the mouth before they're expected, these are the most reasonable explanations. I advise such patients to wear mouth guards at night to prevent the premature aging of their mouths.

Frankly, some people are going to be more prone to bone loss as they age than others. It's not always possible to know who this will be, although genetics could play a role. So if you have any clenching, even in your twenties or thirties, I'd advise you to seriously consider getting a mouth guard. An alternative to this is to get a small injection of Botox in the masseter muscle on the side of the jaw two or three times a year in order to soften it and reduce the kind of clenching that leads to problems later on. I myself habitually clench my jaw when I'm stressed. I first became aware of this when I was in medical school prepping for my examinations. Although I have very good teeth, I began using the masseter injection technique recently on my jaw because of some x-ray findings during my last dental exam. If you think you have an issue with tooth clenching or grinding, I recommend speaking to your dentist about what you could expect to happen to your teeth in the future as a result of this behavior. Very likely, it could lead to unpleasant cosmetic outcomes, and also potentially to medical and health issues.

Volume loss from bone is the main reason why women have such a hard time keeping the area around their mouths looking young. Although many try using fillers and lasers to alleviate the problem, the results are never long-lasting and are sometimes disappointing. Even a facelift will not accommodate for the volume loss from bone tissue in this area. I have seen many women who are still struggling to maintain a youthful mouth area even after multiple facelifts.

In men, changes around the mouth are not as pronounced. Men tend to lose volume on their cheekbones. As a man ages, his prominent cheekbones start to flatten and the skin and other soft tissues start to descend and drape around the jawline and mouth. A man's jaw moves inward, as well; however, the side of the jaw moves outward, adding to the heaviness that is apprehended in an older man's jawline.

Please note that bone loss around the mouth by itself does not make anyone appear elderly; it only makes the mouth appear more aged. An elderly face is acquired when bone remodeling occurs on the middle and upper thirds of the face.

The techniques that I have used to prevent and correct this problem have changed since the approval of Sculptra® Aesthetic, a new facial injection treatment that acts as a collagen biostimulator. This product acts like a filler, mimicking the volume loss from bone and slowing down the aging process. If we can imitate bone volume, then we can recreate a more youthful face. I use Sculptra to create a thick collagen sheath on the bones around the cheeks and mandible. This pushes the muscles and soft tissue envelope outward, resulting in a more vital and youthful face. In addition, I use Sculptra around the bony structures above the upper lip and around the nose to shorten the distance from the nose to the mouth.

I also use diluted Sculptra to thicken the skin above the lip with new collagen. This softens vertical lines above the upper lip and creates more support, thus preventing the lip from rolling into the mouth, as well as making it appear fuller.

Sometimes, I use other fillers or lasers in conjunction with Sculptra to achieve optimal results in this troublesome area. My success with this product has helped me to become the #1 user of Sculptra in the United States.

## THE NEGATIVE VECTORS ⬇⬇

A vector is a quantity possessing both magnitude and direction. It is commonly represented by a directed line segment whose length represents the magnitude and whose orientation in space represents the direction. The simplest way to illustrate a vector is as an arrow connecting two points. In a position versus time graph, a vector that is pointing upward is considered a positive vector, and a vector that is pointing downward is usually considered a negative vector.

Ironically, facial aging can be explained mathematically with vectors—and one does not need to be a rocket scientist to understand the explanation!

As far as we are concerned, any vector that is in agreement with the law of gravity and is pointing downward is a negative vector. As the face starts to deflate and descend, negative vectors are created with magnitudes and directions that comply with the changes that we might expect to see in an older individual. In fact, using digital technology we can plug in some-one's negative vectors to create a true-to-life projected picture of their aging face in the future. A person who wishes to see his or her "future face" can upload a digital photo, answer a few questions about his or her habits and lifestyle and—*voila*—a digital image of that person's future face is produced.

In digital aging, an artist uses a computer program that utilizes mathematical equations to project morphological changes selectively on a youthful photo. In order to create the changes in the photo, the artist employs the same vectors that occur in nature to simulate volume loss from fat and bone. In fact, a computer app called Aging Booth can do this in a matter of seconds.

Understanding the aging process and its correlation with negative vectors can provide cosmetic physicians with valuable rejuvenating information. In other words, *learn to reverse these negative vectors and you will be able to reverse the signs of aging.*

Although there are many surgical approaches to correct negative vectors, volume loss correction is still the most simple and valuable method available. Volume replenishment helps make people appear younger because fat volume and bone thickness create three-dimensional positive vectors in a younger face. Attending to the fat volume is imperative if you want to look younger. We've all seen older people who have had facelifts without getting volume replenishment. They have the postsurgical "old face" of which we've spoken. They did not look any younger or better. They just looked like older people with the additional stigma of having bad facelifts that stretched their skin.

During plastic surgery intervention, a surgeon should closely observe the vector direction of pull in order to avoid an unnatural "trapped in a wind tunnel" look. In addition, because facelifts can be tricky in men and have the potential of feminizing their features, the placement of the incision is particularly important. Facelifts have come a long way. Having moved away from subtractive methods, cosmetic surgeons and cosmetic dermatologists now recognize that the restoration of facial volume is critical for helping people to appear younger. I spend a great part of my day using an armamentarium of fillers to restore or add volume to my patients' faces in order to slow down the "darn clock."

I also educate my patients that it is critical to correct any signs of mid-facial descent, temporal wasting, or jowl formation sooner rather than later. This enables them to tackle the formation of any small negative vectors. People who monitor these small negative changes will usually look at least ten years younger than their chronological ages. It is easier to lift tissue that has moved only two centimeters than tissue that has moved five centimeters. My goal is always to use the smallest intervention possible so that my patients will look entirely natural when they walk out of my office.

## RATIOS: PROPORTIONS

Beauty is not arbitrary. It is based on a complex biological equation of ratios and proportions. Scientists, artists, architects, musicians, psychologists, and philosophers of all eras seem to agree with these ratios and proportions. The ancient Greek mathematicians were the first to notice the ubiquity and appeal of certain ratios and proportions with regard to beauty. Pythagoras (c. 570–495 B.C.E.), for instance, claimed that he had discovered the secret of beauty for the universe. He observed that plants, animals, and minerals grow in precise geometrical ratios.

Euclid (c. 365–300 B.C.E.) provided the first known written definition of this phenomenon in his manuscript Elements. Plato (427–347 B.C.E.) agreed and called this geometrical observation the golden ratio. This mathematical ratio can be applied to just about anything created by humankind or Mother Nature that is considered harmonious or beautiful, including the human face. Studies have revealed that the more closely a face conforms to the golden ratio, the more beautiful it is usually considered. This is true despite ethnicity. When a "beautiful" face is divided into two parts, the relative size of the small part to the big part is the same as the ratio of the big part to the whole.

Does this sound complex and confusing? The same formula has been applied to the proportions of the world's great cathedrals. It also exists in the spiral of a snail shell. It turns out that beauty is much more than what is "in the eye of the beholder." We are programmed by nature to appreciate certain proportions.

It was not until the Renaissance in 1509 when the Italian mathematician, Luca Pacioli (1445–1517), figured out the actual measurement of the golden ratio. The so-called divine proportion is 1:1.618. Leonardo da Vinci (1452–1519), a friend of Pacioli, explored this ratio in the human body and then featured it in many of his paintings. It can be found in every part of the human body—not just the face. And interestingly, it applies to everyone's body, except in cases of deformity.

The notion of the golden ratio has prompted several contemporary scientific studies. They have all proved that there is, in fact, a law that governs beauty. The golden ratio is always present in a face that people generally find aesthetically pleasing. By using golden ratio calipers, you can find the same 1:1.618 ratio all over a face. Furthermore, the more symmetrical a face is, the more the golden ratio can be evidenced among its different features.

Unfortunately, as our faces start to lose their volume, changes begin being seen in the proportions of the faces of even the most beautiful of us. These changes are most pronounced around our mouths. As our faces drop and elongate, the concertina effect becomes imminent. Everything drapes around our mouths due to the loss of their underlying support. The ratio of our upper lips to our chins in a young face is 1/3: 2/3. As we age, this ratio approaches 1:1.

I spend a lot of time educating my patients about ratios, proportions, and volume loss in order to effectively address their concerns about perioral (mouth area) aging. The better their understanding, the better they can practice strategies for age reversal and prevention. As our faces age, we can easily see predictable changes in their proportions due to the negative vectors created by volume depletion.

## SYMMETRY = BEAUTY

As the human embryo develops in the womb, it is programmed to grow on two equal parts around the central axis of the spine. If you draw an imaginary line through the center of the body, one side should resemble the other. This holds true for the face, as well. However, small genetic abnormalities, infections, or prenatal malnutrition may result in an alteration of the facial symmetry and design. This alteration is like a permanent record on our faces, which advertises a defect in our genetic health. Symmetry by contrast advertises the absence of genetic or acquired defects. Therefore, when we're looking for a potential partner for procreation, it is genetically imprinted upon us to start by looking at someone's face, skin, and dentition. We are always subconsciously looking for clues on a person's face. As young people, this is an instinct to ensure that our offspring will have a better chance for survival. As older people, it's an instinct not to have to worry about our mate's own survival.

Interestingly, symmetry corresponds to athletic ability as well as to beauty. Have you ever noticed that most athletes seem attractive? No wonder those quarterbacks in high school seemed to have it all. Studies on athletes have found that those with more symmetrical bodies perform better than those with less symmetrical bodies.

Cultural ideas of beauty create a standard of comparison, and this may cause distress and resentment for those who are not blessed with the attributes that render a person "beautiful." Attractive people are treated differently. Researchers have found that they tend to be offered better jobs and earn more money than average-looking people. Although being perceived as beautiful can also be a burden, being attractive is a genetic advantage that many people hope to pass on to their children.

The major downside to physical beauty is that it comes with an expiration date. As we age and start to lose the fat volume on our faces, we also start to lose the symmetry and proportions that once brought us the admiration of others. It's difficult to experience such loss, especially with today's pressure to stay young and beautiful. Too many people are trying to look like celebrities who appear ageless because they are surrounded by servants who do their hair, makeup, feed them, work them out, and dress them. This has created a huge demand for cosmetic procedures. Of course, most of the people who request procedures are holding themselves to unattainable standards by comparing themselves to airbrushed photographs in magazines or films where cinematographers use a special lens and lighting to disguise the physical flaws of the performers. If, as studies suggest, we will be able to extend our life spans past the century mark in the near future, then there will likely be a corresponding social pressure exerted on each of us to extend the expiration date of our physical attributes, as well.

Since the majority of us exhibit some bilateral facial asymmetry, it is easy to understand why beauty was once considered a rarity and a reason for admiration. Today, with the help of plastic surgery and the armamentarium of fillers and makeups that is at our disposal, we now find beautiful people everywhere. All it takes is a nip and a tuck and a little dab of this or that concoction.

Since symmetry equals beauty, and beauty is the main reason people come to see me, I spend a lot of time educating my patients about facial fat loss and the aging process. The face has multiple fat compartments that age independently from one another; some compartments lose fat at a faster rate, while other compartments retain or even increase their amounts of fat (a phenomenon termed *fat malposition*). As the fat compartments become more discernible as separate entities, the face loses its nice transition from one area to the next, thereby disrupting the symmetry of the face and casting unflattering shadows.

I look great when I look at myself in the mirror of my bathroom, but in the dim lighting of the elevator of my apartment building I look like death, because shadows from the contours of my face are exacerbated. This phenomenon is the result of light bouncing against the skin and showing the areas where change is occurring. My advice is not to use what you see in the mirror as a way to torture yourself. Too much light above and not enough around you can be problematic. We all look much better in sunlight and when the light is shining on us from directly in front of us.

Facial fat depletion and craniofacial skeletal volume loss are the key contributing factors to the progress of facial aging. While doing consultations, I observe the faces of my patients to see where there is asymmetry. I then determine whether the asymmetry is due to the way they sleep, a congenital issue, a trauma, or the natural aging process. With the help of facial fillers, I can restore their symmetry, thereby slowing down the darn clock on their appearance. I find that when my patients restore their volume loss and prevent their faces from shifting downward or sinking in, they are able to keep their youthful features longer.

Many of my patients tell me they feel the most concerned about their nasolabial folds or jowls, and they aren't aware that these lines are caused by fat volume loss. I explain that I never put any type of filler in nasolabial folds or jowls that are the result of volume loss, as this would simply add weight to any skin and tissue that is already coming down. This would only add to the negative vectors that have been formed and speed up their aging process.

A negative vertical vector also pulls on the thin skin of the lower eyelid, causing it to lose its elasticity and crinkle. This is pure physics. Once they are introduced to it, it's not hard for my patients to understand the principle.

Many people believe that Botox is only used to correct or

prevent unwanted wrinkles, but in the right hands Botox can restore facial symmetry. It can also be used in cases of trauma or Bell's palsy, and after surgery to treat facial paralysis.

While the asymmetries of our faces give us our unique appearances, they also advertise our attractiveness and health. Sometimes, a minor correction on the face can make an impressive improvement in someone's looks. For example, we can easily see this in the well-known Simpson sisters. Before Ashley Simpson corrected a minor bump on her nose and decreased the size of the tip of her nose, she was less attractive than her beautiful sister, Jessica Simpson. After her rhinoplasty (cosmetic surgery on the nose), Ashley became, without a doubt, the more beautiful sister.

The nose is an important feature in both the frontal and profile views. No wonder rhinoplasty is the most sought-out facial aesthetic procedure in the world. By changing the negative features of a nose, such as it being oversized, and by preserving the positive features, we can achieve a better aesthetic and harmony with the rest of the face. It is important for the nose, cheeks, and chin to be in balance, proportionally, for someone to have an aesthetically pleasing facial profile.

In Iran, which is considered the nose job capital of the world, they have a saying: "Kill me, but make me beautiful." This says it all. In a country where women have to hide most parts of their bodies under voluminous clothing and veil their faces, showing a petite nose has become all the rage. Genetically, Iranian people tend to have prominent noses. I am sure that this was never a reason for much concern in the past. And honestly, there are many beautiful Iranian women and handsome Iranian men with their natural noses intact. However, due to images from Hollywood, a smaller Westernized nose is the primary feature youngsters, both male and female, are looking to improve cosmetically these days in Iran.

Rhinoplasty has apparently become a common reward in Iran for graduating from high school and passing college entrance exams. This nose reshaping procedure undeniably produces an impressive aesthetic change and if it is done properly complements the rest of their Middle Eastern features, creating an exotic beauty.

The nose has an important role on the face. Being front and center, it determines a person's overall appearance. A disproportionately shaped nose can create an optical illusion of having an underdeveloped chin or detract from the ideal ratios of a beautiful face. This is why a smaller, symmetrical nose is desired.

That being said, a smaller nose in a male face can also distort the ratios and symmetry of the masculine ideal. Many male patients have asked me to inject fillers in their noses to make them look stronger and more masculine. Patients will sometimes do a chin augmentation in conjunction with a nose job to create a better balance of facial features.

Beauty is not arbitrary. It is not just in the eye of the beholder or skin deep, although personal preferences do enter into consideration of what makes someone attractive. As a cosmetic dermatologist, I cannot ignore that beauty is a byproduct of precise mathematical measurements and ratios that humanity has been hardwired to perceive. It is a genetically inherited trait that advertises health, athletic capability, and a better chance for the survival of our offspring.

# CHAPTER 3

# All about Skin

The skin is the largest organ of the human body. Its primary task is to serve as a barrier between the internal organs and the outside world. It also regulates body temperature, protects against invasion by infectious microorganisms, and prevents dehydration. It stores fat, water, and vitamin D, and it excretes and expels toxins and waste materials. The skin is also an indicator of internal disease and helps us with our environmental perception. It covers a surface area of approximately 18.9 square feet (the size of a dining room table), weighs approximately eleven pounds or five kilograms (imagine the heft of a bowling ball), and has an average thickness of 2 millimeters (the thickness of a nickel).

The skin is divided into three layers. The most superficial layer, known as the epidermis, has an average thickness of 0.12 millimeter (the thickness of a page of this book) and is primarily composed of skin cells (keratinocytes), pigment-producing cells (melanocytes), and immunoregulating entities known as Langerhans cells and Merkel cells, which act as sensory receptors. It takes about two weeks to shed skin cells from the body, unless there is a disease, such as psoriasis, that is causing skin cell retention.

The keratinocytes and other skin cells native to the epidermis can be damaged and mutated by ultraviolet (UV) rays from the sun, transforming them into cancerous lesions several decades later. The dark coloration of the skin that we experience after sunbathing is an attempt by the skin to prevent sun-induced mutations of the native cells of the skin.

The dermis is a two-fold-thick, inner layer of the skin consisting primarily of connective tissue, cellular elements, and ground substance (sort of like the glue that holds everything together). It has an average thickness of 1.8 millimeters (the thickness of a quarter). Many important structures are contained within the dermis, including blood vessels, nerves, hair, and glands. The dermis also contains a matrix, or biological mesh, of collagen fibers and elastic fibers that gives the skin its support and elasticity.

Normal, unharmed skin is composed of 80 percent collagen and 4 percent elastic fibers. Collagen fibers act like ropes under the skin and give it strength. The elastic fibers are like rubber bands that are entwined among the collagen fibers to prevent the skin from sagging and wrinkling. In addition to structural proteins (which include collagen and elastic fibers), the skin matrix also needs fillers to provide moisture, mechanical cushioning, and a medium for cell-to-cell communication. The glycosoaminoglycans and proteoglycans are gelatinous, natural fillers that provide the dermis with mechanical support and function as a barrier. Hyaluronic acid is the most important of the glycans because it provides the skin with moisture, regulates tissue repair, contributes to the resilience and suppleness of the skin, regulates the movement of cells and the communication between them, and is intimately involved in the immune and inflammatory responses.

Since collagen and elastic fibers need to be surrounded by water, another type of cells known as fibroblasts, which manufacture collagen, increase the content of hyaluronic acid to make sure that the water content in the dermis is adequate. Hyaluronic acid can hold 1,000 times its weight in water, thus providing the skin with moisture and turgor. Turgor is the degree of elasticity of the skin provided by hydration. After menopause, the levels of collagen in the dermis begin to become depleted. Without as much collagen and elastic fibers the need for the fibroblasts to create hyaluronic acid in the skin matrix is diminished, thus causing the skin to thin, wrinkle, and begin to sag. Men's faces are visibly affected by intrinsic factors around midlife, too. The wrinkles you would see on a man's face mainly come from other factors, which are extrinsic, however; as men typically, historically, have paid less attention to their skin care.

The term *solar elastosis* refers to collagen and elastic fibers that are damaged from chronic sun exposure. When collagen is damaged, its fibers start to unwind and separate. Damaged elastic fibers also undergo a morphological change, changing, as it were, from an elastic rubber band to a hard rubber tire. Afterward, the damaged collagen and elastic fibers form aggregates under the skin, resulting in deep wrinkles, broken blood vessels, and leathery looking skin.

The last layer of the skin is the subcutis, or subcutaneous tissue, which constitutes the largest volume of fat tissue in the body. The thickness of this subcutaneous fat may vary from one area of the body to another. For example, it is thick around the abdomen, but extremely thin on the eyelids. The subcutis provides protection from physical trauma and insulates the body. Fat is formed and stored in this layer, which is also where most of the lipid metabolism for nutrition occurs. This layer is a great reserve source of energy for the human body.

Remember the old adage "You can't judge a book by its cover"? Well, I am here to tell you that, yes, you can. The skin reveals a lot about a person. I can usually tell if my friends or patients have just had a rough night. The skin also gives clues about a person's occupation. For example, people that work outdoors tend to have dark sun damage, leathery skin, precancerous and cancerous lesions, and brown spots. You can also see the same changes in people that leisure outdoors in the sun.

In addition, the skin is a good indicator of internal medical problems and genetically inherited diseases. There are many skin manifestations of internal diseases that can help a physician to properly diagnose and treat illnesses. I remember a nice, beautiful lady who came into my practice because of two red spots on her cheeks. She looked at me and said, "Doctor, I want you to laser off these two red spots on my face. I can no longer cover them up with makeup." She had read about me and the lasers that I use to remove facial blood vessels.

When I used my special magnifying lens to look at the lesion, I saw that there was more to this lesion than the red blood vessels. I immediately turned the cosmetic visit into a medical visit and asked if she had been experiencing any medical problems. She replied, "I have only been suffering from asthma for the last seven years, and I seem to be constantly taking prednisone for my shortness of breath."

After learning that there was no family history of asthma, I became suspicious that something else was going on. I took a biopsy sample of the lesion, and the pathology report came back as sarcoidosis, a chronic lung disease. I asked her to see her internist and to get some radiographic studies of her lungs to see if the cause of her shortness of breath was because of sarcoidosis. The radiographic results showed that she did, in fact, have the disease. I told her that her vanity saved her life. After being misdiagnosed for seven years, she now is receiving treatment and has a better quality of life. She is doing great.

There are many diseases that can be diagnosed by observing changes on the skin, hair, and nails. For example, hepatitis turns people's skin yellow. Some collagen-related vascular diseases, like systemic lupus, may show up first on the skin. Also, nails may turn yellow with certain chronic lung diseases. Our skin alerts us when something inside our body is going wrong. The term *genodermatoses* refers to a large group of inherited single-gene disorders and chromosomal disorders with skin manifestations.

During my residency, I learned about a vast number of rare, but impressive, inherited skin disorders. Whenever one of these patients walked into the training clinic, we were able to tell the name of the disease just by looking at their skin and facial characteristics, even before looking at the other manifestations of the disease. Many of these genetically inherited diseases come with a multitude of serious medical problems and malignancies. If there is a strong family history of any of the serious, well-known genodermatoses, a young couple trying to conceive a family should get genetic counseling and consider adoption or not having children.

The fact is that we all want great skin because we are trying to advertise great genetics, reproductive capability, and good health. Everyone that comes to my practice wants beautiful skin. They invest in laser treatments, chemical peels, microdermabrasion, and cosmeceuticals in order to achieve picture-perfect, flawless skin.

This fascination—bordering on obsession—for beautiful skin is a genetically inherited characteristic that has been scientifically proven to impact the way we judge people, subconsciously, by the look of their skin. In movies, skin type is commonly used to communicate whether a character is the hero or the villain. The villain usually has scars, multiple tattoos, or otherwise imperfect skin. Witches are almost always portrayed with large, unsightly moles on their noses or chins. These cues serve as visual shorthand to let us know that these are bad people.

I remember growing up afraid of people with albinism because they were often portrayed as villains in movies. In fact, over the last fifty years there has been only one movie where I can recall someone with albinism being portrayed as a hero: *Powder.* Since albinism is a rare and peculiar genetic mutation, it commonly invokes fear, surprise, or curiosity in others. People have a tendency to fear anything that is unknown or unfamiliar.

Because of the common portrayal of albinism I am concerned

that young children with albinism are going to be treated unfairly and feel isolated. Uneducated people can be superstitious. One of my colleagues treated people with albinism in Malawi on a recent mission trip to Africa. He informed me that not only were the albinos in the villages there not getting appropriate care for the prevention of skin cancers, but they were also being hunted down, like animals, for their body parts. People mutilate their fingers, hands, and other body parts to create "magical potions" for luck and other superstitious rituals. It horrifies me to know that this is actually happening in contemporary Africa.

I am planning to join this friend and colleague on a mission to bring dermatologists to the Island of San Blas, in Panama, where there is a tribe with the genetic mutation that causes albinism. Since people with albinism have no protection from the sun, living on a tropical island without proper medical care is detrimental to their health.

As I mentioned before, we cannot help having the desire for a skin that is supple and free from wrinkles, blemishes, and lesions. This was the main way that our ancestors advertised their suitability to create healthy babies during the Stone Age. Though we have since evolved intellectually, we still have an instinctual need to survey people's skin to assess their health and reproductive capability.

## PREVENTION

Since unblemished skin seems to be universally desired, it makes sense to do everything possible to nurture and take care of the skin. Whether or not you were born with great skin, it is essential to take care of this organ because of the important physiological roles it plays in your life. Be grateful and honor your skin for all the blessings that it provides you.

I love it when younger patients ask me what they can do to prevent wrinkles and keep their skin looking flawless. The question may seem vain, but a certain degree of vanity is important for our health. If it were not for vanity, there would be a world of toothless people because no one would floss. Studies have shown that people who are vain tend to be healthier than those who don't care about the way they look.

My seventy-two-year old patient Gayle has better skin than most of the thirty-somethings that come to me for consultations. She is a vivid example that with the right skin care protocol, a healthy lifestyle, and treatments to maintain the elasticity and integrity of the skin, anyone can achieve a virtually ageless skin. A virtually ageless skin can be achieved by being rich in collagen and elastic fibers, maintaining an adequate level of skin moisture, and by protecting and nurturing our skin cells.

## FACTORS THAT AGE THE SKIN

The aging of our skin is influenced by intrinsic and extrinsic factors. *Intrinsic aging* is genetically predetermined. We were given an internal clock by the genes of our parents, which determine many of the changes that will happen to our skin as we age. Now, due to the study of the new science of epigenetics, we know that our genetic predispositions can sometimes be altered. Expression of a genetic predisposition can be turned on and off depending on environmental conditions—including the environment of our minds. With age, our skin tends to become drier, thinner, and less elastic, causing normal expression lines to become deeper. In addition, the rate of skin cell shedding slows down, causing the skin to lose its luster as it becomes less efficient at retaining moisture. When our skin loses its thickness and elasticity, it is no longer able to compensate for the volume loss from the underlying tissues. This contributes to the negative vectors that form on an aging face.

All of these changes are more drastic and pronounced in women's skin than in men's skin because of menopause, which can cause a woman's skin to get thin, dry, and crepe paper-like in her fifties. You hardly see a man with very thin skin until he is much older. For this reason, I tell all my female patients in their late twenties to start preparing for menopause immediately by putting collagen fibers and elastic fibers "in the bank." You have to be a *billionaire* of collagen and elastic fibers before you reach menopause! I teach each and every one of my female patients how to generate and collect collagen and elastic fibers so that when the menopause arrives in their late forties and early fifties, they will not experience much change in the elasticity and texture of their skin. Of course, we should never forget that women are beautiful because of the light in their eyes, their humor, their wisdom, and their compassion as much as because of the appearance of their skin. I want to help women feel good.

There are many ways that we can increase our bank accounts of collagen and elastic fibers. I recommend that everyone—male as well as female—uses a retinoic acid or a vitamin A derivative cream at night. When used regularly, the family of retinoic acids will prevent the breakdown of the old collagen and elastic fibers and will help create new ones.

Using lasers and light technology to stimulate and accelerate the increase of collagen and elastic fibers via fibroblast stimulation is another efficient way to increase your collagen bank account. In addition, using fillers that work as collagen-stimulating agents is another easy way to increase the levels of collagen and elastic fibers in the skin.

*Extrinsic aging* of the skin is the most rapid accelerator of all the changes that occur in a mature skin. This is a direct result of a patient's lifestyle and environment. Even if you have inherited fantastic genes, you could still have poor skin by abusing yourself with external factors. The factors known to cause the most skin damage are chronic sun exposure, smoking, and poor nutrition. In addition, we can add the force of gravity, free radicals, and our sleeping position to the list.

*Photoaged* is the term that most dermatologists use to describe skin that is severely wrinkled, leathery, and blotchy. Photodamaged skin also tends to have facial spider veins, freckles, and a rough texture. This occurs over a period of years and is more severe in people with fair complexions. Repeated sun exposure breaks down collagen and impairs the synthesis of new collagen. In addition, the keratinocytes, the cells in the outermost layer of the skin, can get damaged by chronic sun exposure, causing them to become malignant and resulting in different types of skin cancers.

Free-radical aging is well understood these days. The theory states that when free radicals, molecules with only one electron, such as oxygen molecules, become unstable they steal electrons from other molecules, resulting in skin cell damage and the further breakdown of collagen. I like to use the analogy of a fresh-cut apple to describe this process. The peel, which is full of antioxidants, tends to neutralize the free radicals and remains unchanged. However the pulp of the apple starts to get brown within minutes due to the oxidation process caused by free radicals. If you add lemon juice (an antioxidant) to the pulp, it will retard the browning. Apple skin doesn't get brown because it is laden with antioxidants. Another comparable situation is when iron begins to rust. This is also the result of oxidation.

Living in today's highly compromised environment, we are constantly being bombarded by free radicals, especially from eating processed foods, but also by using cellular telephones, which emit low-level radiation. For this reason, I advise all of my patients to use oral and topical antioxidants to neutralize free radicals in order to maintain the health and integrity of their skin and stall the overall aging process of the body. To illustrate this point, I often refer to the disease progeria, a genetically inherited disease that makes children unable to produce metabolic antioxidant enzymes. Children affected with this disease appear to age at an extremely accelerated rate. We'll discuss what kind of antioxidant remedies are the best protection in later chapters.

Smoking cigarettes ages the skin faster than anything we

do besides chronic sun exposure. This was first described in a 1965 study that found that smoking leads to facial alterations in 79 percent of habitually smoking women. The face of a smoker tends to lose its healthy glow, becoming pale with a yellowish-gray hue and accumulating more wrinkles than we'd expect for its chronological age. Beside the other health risks of smoking, you definitely don't want to have a smoker's face.

The nicotine in a cigarette reduces the blood flow through the blood vessels of the skin via vasoconstriction (tightening of the blood vessels), preventing oxygen and nutrients from being delivered to vital organs including the skin. Any tissue that gets insufficient oxygen and nutrients will be starved and may incur irreversible detrimental changes. Over time, the lack of oxygen and nutrients will promote the formation of harmful free radicals that damage skin cells and collagen and elastic fibers.

Nicotine also acts as a diuretic, decreasing the amount of moisture retained by the skin and causing it to dry out. This is why smokers tend to have dry, rough skin. Dry skin creates tiny cracks on the skin acid mantle, making it susceptible to microorganisms such as harmful bacteria, fungi, viruses, and chemical allergens. Since the acid mantle has a slightly acidic pH and is the first line of defense against all elements, smokers with dehydrated skin are more prone to skin infections and have a poor wound-healing capacity.

Smoking uses up the essential nutrients of the skin, such as vitamin A and vitamin C. This is problematic because vitamin A is essential for generating new skin cells to replace those that have died and for maintaining the overall health of the skin. Vitamin C, an unstable water-soluble vitamin that cannot be manufactured by the body, is essential in the creation and preservation of collagen in the skin. A vitamin C deficiency accelerates the breakdown of collagen, causing premature wrinkles. Studies have shown that the body loses about 35 milligrams of vitamin C for every cigarette that is smoked.

The physical act of squinting and pursing one's lips while

smoking, which is necessary to inhale the noxious smoke, also contributes to wrinkle formation. There are many other potentially life-threatening health risks associated with smoking, but the effects on the skin are the most visually tangible. If nothing else moves them to quit, I hope that most of my patients are vain enough to avoid or to quit smoking for the sake of their skin and overall health. According to the Tri-County Cessation Center in New York, there are over 4,000 chemicals in cigarette smoke and at least sixty-nine of these chemicals are known to cause cancer. Smoking is, without a doubt, a toxic process that sooner or later takes its toll and claims much more than a youthful-looking skin.

## LIVE IN HARMONY, LET GO OF FEAR

Staying youthful as you age is an earned privileged. Earning it requires you to maintain harmony of mind, body, and spirit. When we are young, mirrors tend to show us our outer appearance. Later, with the passage of time, mirrors show us our inward self. If you live a life consumed with worries, anger, depression, or any energies from the kingdom of darkness (fear), you will see these etched right on your facial expressions. If you refuse to forgive, or to have compassion or be kind, your bitterness reflects right back at you.

Always remember that the eyes are windows to the soul, so as you look in the mirror your soul is gazing back at you to show you all you were, all you are, and all that you will be. Every day, probably without being aware of it, through your thoughts and actions you are choosing to have a face that is young and beautiful or old and haggard. Choose wisely.

# CHAPTER 4

# The Seven Plagues

*ermatitis* is the medical term used to define any malady of the skin. Although thousands of skin disorders are described in the medical literature, only a few account for most visits to the dermatologist. As a resident, I was told not to look for "zebras" —obscure diseases that are only encountered once in a blue moon—when diagnosing a skin disease, but for "horses." In this chapter, we will discuss the seven most common skin disorders that I see in my practice. These skin conditions are mainly nuisances that do not have a malignant potential.

## ACNE

Nothing ruins my day more than waking up in the morning with a big whopper on my face. Especially now that I work as a dermatologist, people expect me to have clear skin. My skin became acne prone in my mid-twenties, and I have been prone to breakouts ever since. I had hoped that upon reaching my forties this ailment would finally vanish. Unfortunately, that has not been the case. I therefore still use a skin care regimen that is designed for a teenager with acne. I have great skin only because I work hard at it.

Acne is the most common skin disorder seen in my practice. I am regularly either treating active breakouts or the blemishes and scars that are left behind. Acne vulgaris, or common acne, affects 60 to 70 percent of the general population at some point during their lives. It is primarily a disorder of adolescence, affecting 85 percent of all teenagers between 12 and 24 years of age. However, it can affect certain people throughout early adulthood and beyond.

The incidence of this disease is about 3 percent of all men and 12 percent of women (until their mid forties). It is certainly unfair that women have to battle this plague whenever their hormones fluctuate. They tend to experience breakouts during or after pregnancy, during menstrual periods, and again when they are becoming perimenopausal. This usually happens to women who had acne as teenagers, but it can also affect those who have always had a relatively clear complexion.

The prevalence and type of acne vary according to ethnic group. Acne vulgaris is more prevalent in Caucasian individuals. Those of Spanish descent tend to be more prone to cystic acne, which often results in severe scarring. While individuals of African descent have a tendency to develop a comedonal type of acne that is characterized by multiple white heads and black heads that become infected. Hair products that are used for moisturization can exacerbate this condition.

Patients always ask me about the relationship between diet and acne. Although I was taught in my residency that there is no real correlation between diet and breakouts, I tell my patients that if they notice that a particular food product exacerbates the problem, they should avoid it. Personally, I have noticed that whenever I eat too much chocolate, I immediately have a breakout. Although I have not given it up completely, I do eat a lot less chocolate these days.

There is a theory that the caffeine in the chocolate stimulates sebum production, which in turn leads to the formation of microcomedones. In addition, some studies clearly show that dairy products, especially skim milk, can increase the likelihood of breakouts in certain individuals. I ask my patients to humor me for a couple of weeks by cutting out all dairy products to see if there is an improvement. This tactic is often quite successful.

Another common question is if stress causes the skin to break out. Absolutely! Stress always causes any skin condition to get worse—especially acne. When you're stressed, your adrenal gland releases androgens and cortisol. This can cause a chemical imbalance in your bloodstream that leads to breakouts. Exercising, getting sufficient sleep, and setting aside time to meditate or practice a relaxation technique are great ways to relieve stress. In addition, I use aromatherapy and, when all else fails, valerian root, a food supplement that has calming properties.

The cause of acne is multifactorial and has a strong genetic correlation. This means that if both parents in a particular family have had acne, three out of four of their children will be affected with the disease. However, if only one parent had acne, only one out of four of their children are likely to be troubled by this plague. It is important to note that there are always exceptions and variations in the mode of genetic transmission of this disease and not every family will have the same pattern. Acne may even skip some generations.

The development of acne starts with the formation of a microplug in the upper portion of the hair follicle. This occurs when the dead skin cells that are usually shed every two weeks mix with sebum, creating a bottleneck plug that we call a *comedone.* Since comedones are food for bacteria, they tend to get infected and turn into the infamous zits. The more comedones or microplugs that are formed, the greater the likelihood that bacteria will cause an infection. Propionibacterium acnes are the main culprits for most of the acne breakouts that we encounter. The infection itself is not the main problem, but rather the body's inflammatory response to the infection. The type of inflammatory response determines the severity of the breakout and the severity of the discoloration and scarring. The more pronounced the inflammation, the greater the likelihood that there will be abnormal healing.

In order to ensure clear skin, we need to reduce the number of microplug formations and the level of bacteria on the skin. Depending on the type and severity of the acne breakouts, treatment varies from using medicated washes and topical medications to taking oral antibiotics, Accutane® (isotretinoin), or doing hormonal therapy. The introduction of phototherapeutic treatments (for example, special lights and lasers) has also shown promising results in the treatment of mild to moderate acne.

We treat mild to moderate acne with Pore War™ (made by Shino Bay® Cosmetic Solutions). Using a balanced combination of three powerful ingredients to keep the pores clean and unclogged, this citrus wash melts blackheads and whiteheads. In addition I recommend using a topical antibiotic for the morning and a retinoic acid cream or gel for nighttime. Retinoic acids work by normalizing the skin exfoliation around the follicle, thus preventing the formation of comedones. Although there are many retinoic acids on the market, my favorites to combat acne are Differin®, Epiduo®, Retin-A Micro® and Tazorac®. During the day, I prefer topical preparations of benzoyl peroxide alone or in combination with clindamycin antibiotic. My favorites include NeoBenz® Micro, Benzaclin®, and Duac®.

For moderate to severe acne, I usually do the same topical regimen as above, but I tend to add oral antibiotics to the regimen. Minocycline and doxycycline are the most common antibiotics used to treat most acne breakouts. If my patient is female and the breakouts are being caused by a hormonal imbalance, then an oral contraceptive or an anti-androgenic medication may be used to counteract sebum overproduction. I get great results using 25 milligrams of spironolactone once daily for hormone-induced breakouts. For severe acne with inflammation and scarring, the best existing solution is Acutane. There are some people, however, who cannot tolerate this medication because of adverse reactions, or due to drug sensitivity.

Treatments of alternating blue and red lights from light-emitting diodes (LEDs) can be a great option for those who dislike using lotions and potions to treat their acne. In addition, there are various lasers treatments that help minimize breakouts in patients with mild to moderate acne.

As the aftermath of acne breakouts can be as embarrassing and distressing as the breakouts themselves, many of my patients seek my help to minimize their scarring and discoloration. In my practice, we have a plethora of laser treatments that help to minimize scarring and improve skin tone texture. The SmartSkin $CO_2$™ (made by Cynosure, Inc.), a microablative technology for lighter skin types, and the Affirm™ MultiPlex™ Laser (made by Cynosure, Inc.) for darker skin types are the most amazing lasers on the market for improving acne scarring and helping patients achieve a more beautiful complexion.

## ROSACEA

In his play *Henry V,* Shakespeare was one of the first writers to describe the condition now known as rosacea. There are many comical references in the play to the "red face." My favorite is about Bardolph, a character with rosacea, who had a flea land on his red nose. A boy who witnessed the incident said that when he saw the flea stick to Bardolph's nose it looked like a black soul burning in hell. Although it may seem a bit melodramatic, given the heat-like discomfort experienced by those who suffer from the infamous flush of this plague, it is not incredibly off base.

A French surgeon from the fourteenth century, Dr. Guy de Chauliac, was the first to describe the medical condition known today as rosacea. Due to the rosy appearance it gives to the cheeks and nose, it was once considered a disease caused by an excessive consumption of alcohol. Even today, many people get mistaken as alcoholics or drunks because of the prominent redness rosacea causes on their faces.

Rosacea is a long-term inflammatory disease that mostly affects women between the ages of thirty and fifty, as well as people with fair skin. When they do get it, however, men usually have the most severe cases. Rosacea is characterized by inflammatory eruptions on the areas of flushing, as well as demarcated small red blood vessels and enlarged sebaceous glands.

There are different forms of this disease. In the mildest form, known as the flushing type, certain foods, excessive heat, and alcoholic beverages cause someone's face to flush. With time, this may progress to acneiform bumps on the areas of flushing. One severe type of rosacea is characterized by deep-seated cystic lesions, intense redness, and inflammation. Another very disfiguring type, rhinophyma, mainly affects men over forty and causes lobulated permanent lesions on the nose. W. C. Fields has been the poster child for this type of rosacea for decades. Yet another type, ocular rosacea, is characterized by persistent sensations of burning, dryness, redness, and grittiness in the eyes.

The cause of rosacea is debated in the medical community. Some theories propose that microorganisms, such as bacteria, skin mites, and yeast, are possible causes. Others propose that the irritation of follicles by topical agents, sun damage, inflammatory abnormalities, and genetics are the root causes. Although the cause of rosacea is not well understood, the mechanism of action that leads to flushing and inflammatory lesions is better grasped. The flushing is caused by a dilation of the superficial blood vessels of the skin. As with blushing, stress and heightened emotions can worsen the condition. But although this phenomenon is under the control of the nervous system, it is not considered a neurological disorder.

It has been proposed that a small amount of soft plasma leaks from the blood vessels to the skin when dilation occurs.

The white blood cells in the plasma promote an inflammatory response that worsens with the dilation of the blood vessels. The white blood cells are responsible for surveying the body and launching an immunological attack against anything that the body does not recognize as itself. Having higher than usual levels of white blood cells around the skin therefore leads to an extremely vigilant immune system—and extremely sensitive skin.

In my practice, I use a variety of analogies to help my patients understand different disease processes. In the case of rosacea, I ask them to imagine that the superficial blood vessels on their rosy cheeks or noses are like a freeway and that the cars on the freeway (the white blood cells) are doing surveillance. Since these blood vessels are in close proximity to the skin, it is easy for white blood cells to leak out of them and come into contact with irritants in cosmetics, microscopic mites, bacteria, or yeast. The white blood cells, in turn, start an inflammatory response that can lead to redness or small, inflamed puss-filled bumps on the face. For this reason, laser facials that target the blood vessels can often dramatically improve the condition of rosacea. If the freeway that carries the white blood vessels is wiped out, then the inflammatory white blood cells cannot leak out and into the skin.

In order to find the best treatment, a dermatologist first identifies the type of rosacea that a patient presents. Early treatment of this disease is crucial as it becomes more difficult to treat as time progresses. Once the type and severity of rosacea is determined, a dermatologist can use an arsenal of creams, antibiotics, lasers, and surgical treatments to alleviate the disease. There is good news for people with the flushing type of rosacea. Mirvaso® (brimonidine), a topical gel, can restore your skin to a normal tone. It's sort of like a Visine™ for the skin.

In my opinion, lasers are the best treatment for the redness, flushing, and bumpy lesions of rhynophymatous rosacea. In addition, laser treatments tend to decrease and sometimes reverse the cycles of the inflammatory type of rosacea when used in conjunction with more traditional types of treatment, such as topical and systemic antibiotics.

## ECZEMA

Although the term *eczema* seems to have originated from the Greek word *ekzein,* mentioned in literature for the first time in 543 c.e., I can assure you that the use of Windex®, as seen in the 2002 comedy film *My Big Fat Greek Wedding,* has no basis as a remedy for this condition. The actual meaning of the word eczema is "to boil out," and it is suggestive of the red bumps and blister-like lesions that emerge from the skin. Eczema causes intense itchiness and discomfort that eventually turns into thick, plaque-like patches of dry skin.

The term *eczema* is widely used to describe a variety of medical conditions that lead to inflamed or irritated skin. There are multiple forms and subtypes of this condition. Some of the most common types include atopic dermatitis, dyshidrotic eczema, nummular eczema, hand eczema, and winter eczema.

Eczema usually has a genetic component and is commonly seen in what we consider to be an atopic family—one with a history of allergies, asthma, and eczema. I had asthma as a child. Later, around my mid-thirties, I developed eczema. I tell my patients that eczema is like having asthma in their skin. The cells that contribute to an asthma attack are the same culprits that seem to boil out of the skin during an eczema breakout.

It is important for patients with eczema to understand the disease and to make some minor, but very important, changes at home. For example, they should use a mild cleanser without perfume or colorants when bathing, and keep showers to a maximum of ten to fifteen minutes. Additionally, all towels, sheets, and clothing should be washed with perfume and dye-free detergents. Fabric softeners and drying sheets should be avoided.

Moisturization is essential for maintaining a good skin barrier and for managing and relieving the itchiness and burning associated with eczema. Products like Cerave®, Cetaphil®, and Aveeno® Eczema Therapy are great moisturizers for eczematous skin. When the skin is extremely dry and sensitive, I advise my patients to use Aquaphor® ointment or Crisco® All-Vegetable Shortening to repair their skin barriers.

There are a multitude of different prescribed creams, ointments, and lotions that I use to treat active eczema breakouts. I choose them according to the patient's age, the location of the breakout on their bodies, and the severity of the disease. There are many new products on the market that are steroid-free which can help maintain a healthy skin by increasing its moisture content.

Extreme cases of atopic dermatitis or eczema may require the intervention of systemic medications and other methods to regulate the immune system and to alleviate some of the symptoms. Some cases are so severe that patients have to be hospitalized; fortunately, these cases are not common.

It is imperative that all eczema patients follow the aforementioned at-home recommendations for shower soaps, detergents, and moisturization to maintain a healthier skin and to prevent relapses.

## WRINKLES

Coco Chanel once said: "At age fifty we get the face that we deserve." After thinking about this statement, I concluded that if I ever got tired of injecting Botox into my face, I would do everything in my power to develop only those wrinkles associated with laughter and compassion. Later in my life I want to have a sweet face, not a grumpy old man's face!

Many people believe that they can tell a lot about a person's character by the lines on his or her face. If you have the "number 11" lines between your eyebrows, you probably worry a lot. If you have crow's feet, it's a sign that you smile a lot, making you a more approachable and joyful individual. By contrast, lines around the mouth are caused by frowning and show a gloomy personality.

Many patients tell me that they are generally very happy and friendly, but the lines between their eyebrows paint a different story. As a result of the groove marks, they often feel that people are not reading them correctly. This is precisely when a little Botox can turn things around.

If I am a happy-go-lucky person and I get a grumpy old man's face, what have I done to deserve that? It does not seem fair! The truth is that it has to do with our facial anatomy and our genetics, as much as with external aging factors such as sun damage and smoking cigarettes. Nevertheless, if you are constantly making the same facial expressions, over time you will acquire wrinkles that are perpendicular to the muscles of your facial expressions.

Wrinkles tend to occur in the areas of the face where we make a lot of expressive movements. The muscles responsible for our facial expressions create continuous tension in the skin of the face and the neck. Over time, this tension causes the architecture of the collagen and elastic fibers, which keep the skin looking supple and wrinkle free, to become rearranged.

In Chapter 3, I enlightened you about collagen and elastic fibers. Since we are talking about wrinkles, it is important to understand that while most cells in the human body are constantly dying and replicating, collagen and elastic fibers are not. Fibroblasts, the cells that create collagen, are replaced approximately every thirty years. Therefore, we naturally break down more collagen and elastic fibers than we can generate. This is a part of the natural aging of the skin, as well as an intrinsic factor.

Many environmental, or extrinsic, factors, such as smoking and sun exposure, also contribute to the acceleration of the breakdown of existing collagen and elastic fibers. This invariably leads to an increase in the number of deep wrinkles and the sagging of the skin.

In my practice, we have different methods to prevent and correct premature aging of the skin and wrinkle formation. We can achieve this, mechanically, by injuring the skin with a laser light that destroys the broken-down collagen and elastic fibers and replaces them with new ones. Another mechanically effective method is a microneedling technique in which a roller with tiny needles is rolled over the face to create trauma. We can achieve a similar result, chemically, by using poly-L-lactic acid (sold as Sculptra) to induce the formation of new collagen fibers. Another inexpensive method is to use cosmeceuticals that contain retinoic acid or any other molecule that promotes the formation of new collagen and elastic fibers.

I recently met Pat, an eighty-one-years young lady who has no wrinkles and looks thirty years younger than her chronological age. She learned at an early age how to avoid the ravishing effects of the intrinsic and extrinsic factors that cause the skin to age. She gives all of us hope and inspiration because it shows us that anyone can have beautiful skin at any age. I have always bragged about the perfect skin of my friend Joan (age seventy-six at the time of this writing), but then Pat came along and took the title for having beautiful skin at any age.

## SCARS

Scars, or cicatrices, are entities on the skin that always tell a story. Most of the time we can vividly recall the events by which we acquired them. During a traumatic event, the structure and lattice of the skin, deep down to the dermis, are ruptured. The body then goes into high gear to heal the injured tissue, since having an open wound could potentially lead to an infection. The fibroblast cells in the skin lay down new collagen and elastic tissue in such a hurry that they often do not match the rest of the skin in texture and tone. For this reason, a scar looks and feels different than the surrounding, normal skin.

Most skin scars are flat, pale, and leave a mark that resembles the original injury that caused them. However, there are some scars that tend to get thicker or extend outside the area of injury. We see this with hypertrophic scars and keloids, respectively. These types of scars are the result of too much production of collagen in the wound. Alternatively, atrophic scars appear to have very little skin tissue in them. A perfect example of an atrophic scar can be appreciated in stretch marks. Stretch marks, usually acquired during pregnancy, are superficial scars that occur when the tissue under the skin grows faster than the skin can accommodate, causing the skin to rip.

Hypertrophic scars are usually raised, reddish, and confined to the wound margin. They are often painful or itchy, and they can be managed with silicon sheets, intralesional steroids, or lasers. With time, they also have the tendency to get better on their own.

Keloids tend to extend beyond the wound margin and may be symptomatic. They slowly form after the lesion has completely healed and are very difficult to treat. The rate of recurrence for keloids is high, causing frustration for both the patient and the treating physician. They can occur in anyone, but are more common in dark-skinned individuals. Unlike hypertrophic scars, keloids can grow indefinitely into large tumors. The areas of predilection for keloid formation are usually on the chest, back, and shoulders.

In our clinic we use a pulsed dye laser to prevent scar formation after surgery and also to treat recently formed scars. For mature or hypertrophic scars, we use either the Affirm MultiPlex Laser or the SmartSkin $CO_2$ (made by Cynosure, Inc.) to get phenomenal results. In addition, we have successfully improved—and even eliminated—some keloids with the Affirm MultiPlex Laser in combination with intralesional injections. It is very exciting that we can now actually treat keloids, as they have been frustrating the medical community for years.

Most scars treated with lasers blend very well with the surrounding normal skin. Although they can sometimes blend so well that they are hardly visible, scars are never 100 percent removed.

## MELASMA

Commonly known as the "mask of pregnancy," melasma is a discoloration of the face that tends to occur during gestation. Although the cause of this disease is poorly understood, we do know that it is correlated with a hormonal imbalance and exposure to sunlight. It is found mostly in women of Asian and Hispanic origin. However, people from other ethnic groups, such as Native Americans, Germans, Russians, and those of Jewish descent, are also afflicted with this plague. The incidence of melasma also increases in patients with thyroid disease and for those taking birth control pills or hormone replacement medications.

Melasma presents as dark, irregular patches on the cheeks, nose, lips, and forehead. The patches appear slowly and become both darker and larger over time. Although this condition can be diagnosed visually quite well, a wood's lamp or black light may be needed to discern if the patient has dermal melasma, a type that is much more difficult to treat.

My practice is in Fort Lauderdale, Florida (aka the Sunshine State), so you can imagine how many cases are presented in my office every day. Not only do we have a year-round outdoor lifestyle, we also have a large Latino community. As a result of the cases that I have seen, I have learned much about this plague. Except for dermal melasma, I have always been able to alleviate melasma fairly quickly; however, the rate of recurrence is high. I ask my patients all the time if they are protecting themselves from the sun. They all respond with a big "Yes!" and then go on to say, "Doctor, I use SPF 50 every morning!"

I later discovered that most of these patients mistakenly believed that using a high SPF sunscreen in the morning would protect them for the entire day. So I had to educate them about the necessity of reapplication. In the process, I realized that reapplying lotion throughout the day was a nearly impossible task for them. Working women with melasma tend to wear makeup to cover up the dark patches. No woman in her right mind will put sunscreen over her makeup every two hours to ensure that she is protected from sunlight. I was as frustrated about this dilemma as my patients. The solution, however, was right in front of my eyes. I personally use a powdered sunscreen called Sunforgettable® (made by Colorescience) because I have acne-prone skin. This is a physical sunscreen that protects the skin from UVA and UVB a bit longer than cream chemical sunscreens. Now I advise all my clients to use this product or something similar.

Since women already tend to reapply pressed powder to freshen up their makeup, I figured that using the powder sunscreen would be a user-friendly alternative for women. It helped ensure that my melasma patients could be protected from the sun at all times. Now, if they are at work and someone asks them to go across the street to get lunch, all they have to do is take their powder sticks out of their purses and reapply powder. Believe it or not, since I have been recommending powder sunscreen for reapplication, the recurrence rate of melasma in my office has diminished significantly. Sun protection is truly the first step to start treating this condition. In the next chapter, you will learn all there is to know about sun protection and photo damage.

Our treatment of melasma varies with the type (dermal vs. epidermal), the severity, and its resistance to conventional treatments. It can be treated with preparations of hydroquinone alone or with a mixture of hydroquinone and other melanin inhibitors, such as kojic acid, licorice, or glycolic acid. Chemicals peels and laser treatments are also available.

I usually treat melasma with a 4-percent hydroquinone cream that is used nightly. If this treatment fails to alleviate the discoloration, I use a more aggressive treatment from the Affirm MultiPlex Laser, which has a 1440-nanometer (nm) wavelength.

A nanometer is a unit of length in the metric system that's equal to one-billionth of a meter. It is important to treat melasma with long-wavelength lasers because short-wavelength laser light can worsen the condition. After the laser treatment, patients use a hydroquinone and tretinoin cream mixture, such as Tri-Luma® or Cosmelan® MD or Melanage Peel® (made by Young Pharmaceuticals), to accelerate the vanishing of the discoloration.

There is no cure for melasma. For some women, it can take months or years before we see real improvement; for others, it is a chronic dilemma. Once it resolves or improves, I advise my patients to continue with a maintenance regimen. The biggest mistake that women with this condition make is to think that they are cured after it seems gone. They become careless about sun and light protection, and then it all comes back with a vengeance. In order to prevent a rebound, we offer a maintenance kit to inhibit tyrosinase, an enzyme necessary to make brown pigment. We recommend our proprietary formula of N-lighten Me™ (made by Shino Bay™ Cosmetics). It's a moisturizer with tyrosinase inhibitors and a 2-percent hydroquinone plus kojic acid gel or Lytera® Skin Brightening Complex (made by SkinMedica).

It is also important to know that sunlight is not the only way to activate pigmentation in melasma. There are some types of artificial lighting that can also stimulate pigment formation. I advise some of my most difficult patients to use powdered sunscreen even while watching television at night so that they may protect themselves from all sources of light exposure. Although it may seem tedious, this recommendation tends to be effective. Dermal melasma is extremely difficult to treat and has a high recurrence rate. Products containing mandelic acid have been shown to be somewhat effective with this type of melasma. However, until we better understand this disease, it is going to be a bit frustrating for both the patient and the treating physician.

## BLEMISHES

Most of us are forever dreaming to achieve a flawless complexion. Whenever there is a little bump, mark, or discoloration on our skin, we immediately feel tainted. As a dermatologist, I spend a great part of my day helping my patients to achieve a complexion that is luminous, supple, and devoid of blemishes.

By definition, blemishes are marks or discoloration on the skin, such as blackheads, age spots, and freckles. As with port wine stains and other skin discolorations, these can be inherited. Most blemishes on our skin are either red or brown. Blemishes that are red have a vascular component, while those that are brown contain melanin.

Brown spots can be acquired during inflammation, such as after an acne breakout or a trauma to the skin. The more pronounced the inflammation, the darker the discoloration. This type of brown discoloration is called postinflammatory hyperpigmentation. The darker the skin type, the darker the discoloration—and the longer it will take to vanish. A preparation of 4-percent hydroquinone acts as a bleaching agent and tends to alleviate most blemishes. However, for people like me, who are sensitive to this product, the hydroquinone preparations can actually cause the skin to get darker. The product becomes an irritant to the skin, generating inflammation that can add even more pigment to a blemish.

I tend to use a glycolic acid preparation of mandelic acid or kojic acid for these individuals. The fastest way to help post inflammatory blemishes is by using a 1064-nm wavelength laser (known as a Nd:YAG laser) every two weeks combined with a bleaching agent or glycolic acid preparation at home.

Other common types of acquired brown blemishes are sun-induced freckles and age spots. These tend to occur years after chronic sun exposure. As a joke, I usually refer to these blemishes as "signs of getting younger" or "payback time spots." When I moved to the United States from Panama at seventeen,

I stopped going out in the sun and began protecting my skin constantly. Even so, when I turned forty it was payback time for me. The skin on and around my nose started to develop dark brown age spots and I was distressed to see the emergence of those unsightly blemishes.

The truth is that the majority of our sun damage is acquired before we are twenty years old. It can take decades for us to see the repercussions of the unprotected sun exposure on our skin from when we were teenagers or younger.

There are several treatments to ameliorate sun-induced blemishes. Using bleaching or lightening agents has led to a degree of success, in most cases. However, some of these brown blemishes can be very resistant to topical treatments. In our practice, we use a 755-nm wavelength alexandrite laser to get rid of sun-induced brown spots in only one session. It is very important to understand that not all brown, sun-induced spots are age spots. Lentigo malignant, which can resemble an age spot, is a superficial melanoma that has the potential to be lethal if not caught early enough. Only a properly trained physician is qualified to discern whether a brown spot in question is benign or if it requires immediate attention.

Red blemishes can be the result of inflammation, as we see after acne breakouts in individuals with light-skinned complexions or in newly formed stretch marks and hypertrophic scars. Most of them eventually turn into white and glossy looking scars over time. There are many creams, gels, and silicon sheets that can alleviate the discoloration and improve the final scar. However, the best treatment for these types of lesions is the 585–595-nm wavelength pulsed dye laser. This vascular laser takes advantage of the bright red coloration of these lesions to treat them. The heat generated under the skin helps remodel the collagen in the scar, stimulating collagen that is more compatible with the rest of the skin. This causes the scar to blend to the point of sometimes being almost invisible to the naked eye.

There are other red blemishes on the skin that may be acquired or for which someone may have a genetic predisposition, such as broken capillaries on the face, hemangiomas, spider veins, and port wine stains. The best way to treat them is with vascular lasers whose wavelengths have an affinity for red lesions. We use a double laser treatment, or multiplex technology, along with the Cynergy™ laser (made by Cynosure, Inc.), which combines the 585–595 nm pulsed dye laser with the 1064 nm Nd:YAG laser. These two wavelengths have an affinity to the hemoglobin in the blood vessels, making them ideally suited to eliminate red blemishes on the face. There are other light systems, like the intense pulsed light (IPL), that are also very effective in the removal of sun-induced brown spots. I tend to use this device when the brown spots are diffuse and cover a large surface area.

We'll explore laser treatments, such as these, in depth later in the book.

# CHAPTER 5

# Something about Mary

Who can forget the sleeper hit from 1998 with Cameron Diaz, *There's Something about Mary?* Many scenes still make me laugh though I've watched the movie several times. In my practice, when I say, "There is something about Mary," everyone knows exactly what I am referring to: Mary's sun-worshipping and unnaturally tan neighbor, Magda. Not only is she one of the most memorable characters in the movie, she's also caused many sunbathers to rethink their sun-adoring habits.

I live in South Florida where it's bright and hot most of the year. People move here for the year-round sun and outdoor lifestyle. Unfortunately, fictitious characters like Magda are far too real in our communities. I see so many beautiful men and women with deep brown, leathery skin and premature wrinkles. It always makes me wonder, *Do they see what I see? Do they really think that they look great? Do they care about getting skin cancer or about premature aging?* When asked, many say that they look and feel better when they have a tan. I hear all kinds of comments: "I feel unattractive being pasty white," "I look thinner with a tan," And "I feel depressed if I don't get enough sun." It seems they have set aside the health consequences in order to feel good about themselves.

Adoration of the sun is nothing new. Four hundred years ago, in *Antony and Cleopatra,* Shakespeare wrote a line for one of the most beautiful women of history—and the original bombshell—Cleopatra. Comparing how she feels when her lover is away to the effects of sun exposure, she says:

*Think on me,*
*That am with Phoebus' amorous pinches black,*
*And wrinkled deep in time*

Phoebus was the ancient Egyptian sun god. That Shakespeare could pen these lines indicates that even 400 years ago, everyone knew that the sun causes most of the wrinkles on our skin. Nevertheless, it does not change the fact that those "amorous pinches of the sun" make us feel great.

It is a fact that we need to receive at least fifteen minutes of sunlight a day over approximately 25 percent of our skin to stimulate our bodies to create vitamin D. An insufficiency in vitamin D appears to increase the risk of several cancers, including breast cancer and colon cancer. It is also associated with an increased incidence of diabetes, high blood pressure, multiple sclerosis, and osteoporosis. However, please do not misinterpret this as a mandate to go bake in the sun for hours in order to make vitamin D!

Statistically, one in five Americans will develop skin cancer during his or her lifetime. Approximately one million new cases of skin cancer are diagnosed every year, and one person dies of melanoma every sixty-two minutes in the United States. I would never tell my patients not to enjoy being outdoors or getting some sun, but I do want them to be cautious and smart about it. Therefore, I assist all my patients in developing a comprehensive sun protection program for being outdoors. I tell them to schedule their outdoor activities either before 10:00 A.M. or after 4:00 P.M., when the sun's rays are least intense. In addition, I recommend using a broad-spectrum sunblock or sunscreen with a sun protection factor (SPF) 30 or above, seeking shade whenever possible, and wearing protective clothing and sunglasses.

The sun emits three different types of rays that reach the surface of the Earth: visible, ultraviolet, and infrared. These rays are placed into different categories according to their wavelengths. The wavelength is simply the distance from the sun to the Earth measured in nanometers (nm).

Visible light corresponds to wavelengths that emit colors detectable by the human eye. The visible colors (ranging from shortest to longest wavelength) are violet, blue, green, yellow, orange, and red.

Energy from shorter wavelengths that is "bluer" than blue and cannot be seen by the human eye is called ultraviolet light. Since ultraviolet light is colorless, the only way we know that it exists is because we get sunburned without sun protection.

Ultraviolet light is divided into three rays with different wavelengths. Ranging from shortest to longest wavelength, these are: UVC, UVB, and UVA. UVC, the shortest wavelength from the sun, does not usually reach the surface of the Earth because most of it is absorbed by the ozone layer. In theory, prolonged exposure to UVC is considered harmful and can even be fatal. Increased exposure to UVC rays is one of the main reasons that many scientists are concerned about the depletion of the ozone layer.

UVB rays are responsible for most sunburns and skin cancers, and for the tanning response of sunbathers' skin. This wavelength is only capable of penetrating to the level of the skin's epidermis. It stimulates the melanocyte cells to produce melanin, or brown pigment. The amount of burning UVB rays in our sunlight varies by season, the time of the day, and our location. This is one of the reasons why I recommend that my patients do most of their outdoor activities during the times of the day when the UVB rays are the weakest. In Florida, where I have my practice, the UVB rays are intense.

UVA is the longest wavelength emanating from the sun. Although UVA rays are far less capable of inducing sunburns than UVB rays, dermatologists and scientists agree that it is the most damaging to the body of any of the sun's rays and most responsible for noticeable photoaging. Furthermore, although not previously thought to be as photocarcinogenic as UVB, recent studies suggest that UVA also plays a role in the development of skin cancers. This wavelength penetrates deeply into the skin, down to the level of the dermis. UVA rays are always the same, regardless of the time of the day or year, meaning that they are just as harmful to the skin in January as they are in July.

Though UVA rays are far less capable of causing sunburns than UVB rays, a combined study by Australian and U.S. researchers recently showed that UVA radiation is more carcinogenic than UVB rays. Prolonged exposure to UVA rays cracks and shrinks the collagen and elastic fibers, leading to solar elastosis (wrinkled, photodamaged skin). In addition, the blood vessels may become permanently dilated, causing the skin to have a permanently flushed hue. Since they penetrate deeply into the skin, UVA rays can also destroy melanocyte cells, leaving confetti-like white spots all over the skin. They can cause melanocyte cells to become hyperactive and create brown spots (senile lentigos), one of those "signs of getting younger" that we previously discussed.

In summary, the sun's ultraviolet rays injure the DNA of the skin's epidermal cells, triggering a natural protective mechanism in which specific enzymes come to the rescue of the skin cells' DNA to try to repair the damage. However, if the unprotected sun exposure continues, the enzymes can no longer repair the DNA successfully, which can lead to skin cell mutations, and eventually, skin cancer.

Energy from very long wavelengths that is "redder" than red and cannot be seen by the human eye is called infrared light. The only reason that we know that infrared light exists is because we can feel the heat from the sun when we are outdoors. A big reason why people often get sunburned on an overcast or cloudy day is that since the clouds absorb a big portion of the infrared wavelengths they do not feel the heat from the sun and believe that it's not possible to get sunburned. However, people have a false sense of security, for although ultraviolet rays cannot be seen or felt, they can travel through the clouds.

Exposing the skin to ultraviolet light, whether from the sun or from tanning beds, has short-term and long-term effects. The short-term effects are immediately visible and include sunburn, blistering, and tanning. The long-term effects from chronic exposure to UV rays, although not visible at first, become evident a few decades later when the skin begins to show signs of photoaging, discoloration, and pre-malignant and malignant lesions.

I grew up in Panama City, Panama, where proximity to the Equator makes the sun brutally strong. I remember getting terrible sunburns walking the several miles distance to go to and from school. On one occasion, I was almost hospitalized for sun poisoning symptoms, including nausea, fever, rapid pulse, headaches, dizziness, and extreme fatigue. After that incident, I avoided the sun like the plague! Fortunately, I became a dermatologist and learned how to tackle these sun-induced nuisances.

## SUNSCREEN

Sun protection is an efficient way to help stop the darn clock and to maintain the health and vitality of the skin. As a dermatologist, it is my duty to educate all my patients about the proper use of sunscreen and adequate protective clothing to prevent premature aging and skin cancer. Most people are confused about sunscreen and what level of sun protection factor (SPF) they should be using. With so many products on the market, the confusion is certainly understandable.

In previous nomenclature, there were both sunblocks and

sunscreens. Now, by FDA regulation there are no more "sunblocks." The kind of products formerly considered sunblocks are opaque formulations that protect the skin by absorbing, reflecting, or scattering up to 99 percent of the UVB and UVA rays we're exposed to. Most of these types of sunscreen contain titanium dioxide, zinc oxide, or a mixture of these two ingredients. In general, products like these are great because of their capability to block out most of the UV spectrum. Most people don't like to use them, however, because they can be messy and leave you looking chalky and ghost-like. Fortunately, new micronized formulations using such ingredients are now available that are much more user friendly.

I personally use a micronized formulation of zinc oxide and titanium dioxide powder sunblock from Colorescience as part of my wrinkle-prevention armamentarium. Sunscreens in this category are my choice for preventing wrinkles because they block out the deeply penetrating UVA rays that tend to damage the skin's collagen and elastic fibers. In addition, they are great for individuals with sensitive skin, since they rarely cause skin irritations or allergic reactions.

By definition, sunscreens are chemicals that act as filters to shield the skin by absorbing specific wavelengths in the range of UV light (200–400 nm). Most sunscreens are composed of a variety of active ingredients, because no single chemical ingredient can block the entire UV spectrum. Some formulations of sunscreen contain a mixture of multiple chemicals, with each one absorbing a region of the UV light spectrum. Still the majority of these chemicals are only able to screen out the burning UVB rays.

Since UVA rays can also injure the skin and cause premature aging, like UVB rays, it is important to choose formulations that also contain chemicals that can screen out UVA rays, such as avobenzone (also known by the trade name Parsol 1789), oxybenzone, and methyl anthranilate. Although sunscreens may be more cosmetically elegant than sunblock, it is important to remember to reapply sunscreen every two hours to avoid getting sunburn. Using a water-resistant formulation is ideal for people who are involved in water sports or for individuals who tend to sweat a lot.

Choosing a good sunscreen means much more than just deciding on an SPF factor or choosing between a cream, powder, or spray. The SPF number only tells us how much of the sun's UVB rays can be screened out by the product. A sunscreen user can determine how long the product is going to be effective by simply multiplying the SPF figure listed on the package by the length of time it usually takes to get sunburn without sunscreen protection. For example, if someone usually develops sunburn after 10 minutes of sun exposure without any protection, a sunscreen or sunscreen of SPF 15 will protect this individual for 150 minutes (15 multiplied by 10).

Obviously, this can only be true if the right amount of product is applied and reapplied as directed. In my opinion, everyone should use a daily sunscreen that is at least SPF 15, which screens out about 93 percent of the UVB rays. This advice is appropriate even for people who rarely go outdoors, but who frequently sit near windows and are exposed to natural sunlight, or who often drive in cars. There is a famous photograph printed in dermatology textbooks that shows a woman who is more aged on one side of her face than the other. Having worked near a window for twenty years, the left side of her face—the side nearest the window—is wrinkled with brown spots. The other side of her face has none.

Drivers of motor vehicles often experience more rapid aging on the left side of their faces, necks, and arms because of their frequent exposure to sunlight. In countries where drivers steer from the right side of the car or truck, the opposite side is affected. A year of casual, unprotected daily sun exposure is equivalent to two full days of baking on the beach without protection.

Sun protection is especially important for people who live in sunny areas and for those who are serious about preventing the premature aging of their skin.

Almost no one applies sunscreens in the same manner as they were applied during SPF testing. Therefore, users do not get full advantage of the SPF figure listed on the package. For a more than adequate coverage of the face and neck, an adult should apply an ounce (about two tablespoons) of sunscreen. In addition, I also tell my patients that they are only getting about half of the advertised SPF, since no one is actually measuring two tablespoons of the product. For this reason, using a higher SPF figure is advisable.

I have also heard the misconception from some of my patients that if you apply a lotion with SPF 30 on top of a lotion with SPF 15, then you will be getting SPF 45. This clearly illustrates the amount of confusion that exists about SPF. Allow me to put this misconception to rest: Layering SPF 30 over SPF 15 actually will give you SPF 25, as the higher SPF gets diluted by the additional ingredients in the other SPF formula. The common misconception has it backward.

For people who spend a lot of time under the sun because of their occupations or recreational activities, SPF 30, which blocks about 96.7 percent of the UVB burning rays, is recommended. Remember to reapply the sun protection every two hours if you are planning to be under the sun for most of the day. Unfortunately, most people are not aware that the sun protection provided by chemical sunscreens is significantly reduced after two hours. For this reason, I promote the use of opaque sunscreens (the kind that were formerly known as sunblocks) because they are more efficient in blocking UV rays. They also tend to protect the skin for a lot longer than chemical-based sunscreens. Also make a point to wear a hat and sun-blocking eyewear.

Another common misconception is that a higher SPF will allow you to stay outdoors for a longer amount of time. For example, many of my patients think that using SPF 30 means that they can be under the sun for double the time of a person using SPF 15. But this isn't true.

Honestly, although any product with an SPF 30 or higher will cost you more, it won't provide a significant increase in the amount of sun protection. For this reason, the Food and Drug Administration (FDA) no longer allows manufacturers to make claims of higher than SPF 50 in the United States.

Sunscreens should be applied approximately thirty minutes prior to going out in the sun. This allows enough time for the skin to absorb the product. It also prevents it from being washed off by perspiration or during water sports. I urge my patients to read the list of ingredients to see how much UVA protection a product offers and ensure that there are no ingredients in it that may cause them an allergic reaction. The way people find out which ingredients cause them to react is that they have a bad experience, and then get a patch test to find out which chemical in the product was responsible.

We humans are organisms that use solar energy as a catalyst for many beneficial metabolic processes in our bodies. We are designed to be outdoor creatures. However, too much of a good thing can also be detrimental for the body. For a healthy body, everyone should get the proper amount of sunlight—ten to fifteen minutes three times a week over 15–25 percent of the skin's surface—but we should also avoid getting sunburns or skin cancer in the process.

Recently, the FDA has taken steps to educate consumers about the effectiveness of sunscreen products and how they work, including the requirement of better labeling of products to ensure that consumers are not being misled by false claims. One such step has been to disallow the claim on labels of *sunblock* as a characteristic of any sun protection product. Companies must instead use the term *sunscreen*. Furthermore, manufacturers can no longer claim their products to be *waterproof* or *sweat proof*. Instead the companies must use the terms *water resistant* and *sweat resistant*. They also must explain on the label for what duration the resistance will last.

# CHAPTER 6

# Through the Years

Coco Chanel once said, "Nature gives you the face you have at twenty. Life shapes the face that you have at thirty. But at fifty, you get the face that you deserve." I absolutely agree. What you do to your skin in your twenties greatly affects how you look in your forties and fifties. In other words, if you don't like the way your skin looks at fifty, it's probably because you abused or neglected it in your twenties. The lines on your face may be caused by genetics, but they also tell the kind of person you are: revealing if you've lived a troubled life or spent too much time in the sun. We earn every single wrinkle and brown spot that we see on our faces.

It is important to understand the requirements of our skin throughout the decades in order to avoid being deficient in the ground substances and elements that help us to maintain a youthful looking face and skin.

## YOUR SKIN IN YOUR TWENTIES

During my high school years I never had a single pimple on my face. Then, during college, I started to break out—horribly. I wished that I'd had acne back when most of my high school classmates were going through it. In this period of my life, I was able to experience, firsthand, what acne can do to someone's self-esteem and confidence. Besides going to school, I was also working as a model, in an era before Photoshop, so having severe breakouts was dreadful and stressful. Using makeup to hide the blemishes during shows aggravated the problem even more. I felt hopeless and depressed.

I wish that I had known back then how to take care of twenty-something skin. It is amazing how even a single pimple could dictate how I felt about my life. The experience helped me to become a more sympathetic and compassionate dermatologist. Thank heaven that, for the most part, acne starts to subside for most people during their twenties.

The most common skin problems we face during our twenties are oiliness and stress-induced breakouts. Stress releases cortisol and others hormones that cause breakouts. There is also evidence that a gradual disappearance of facial baby fat occurs around our twenties. As the fat layer under the skin starts to thin out, the face loses its roundness and softness, and fat is now left in strategic places to hold the face up.

The great thing about this age is that our wrinkles and creases vanish the moment that we relax our faces. The abundance of collagen and elastic fibers recoils the skin back to its beautiful, supple state.

During your twenties, skin cell production slows down, so you begin to get a buildup of dead cells that are incapable of retaining moisture or reflecting light as effectively as in the past. Unless you have oily or acne-prone skin, the complexion loses some of its luster and becomes a bit dry and dull. Sun-induced freckles may begin to appear, and the pores may become enlarged. This is also when a few signs of the things to come from our days spent in the sun start to manifest.

As you can see, nature gives us the skin and faces that we have in our twenties, just like Coco Chanel said.

In this decade, it is imperative that everyone become serious about sun protection. You must avoid smoking and second-hand smoke. Using an oil-free moisturizing lotion can be helpful as long as the skin is not oily or acne prone. In addition, try to train yourself to sleep on your back to avoid fat cell volume depletion or making a permanent skin impression on your face. When you are reaching the end of your twenties, it would be a great idea to introduce a retinol moisturizing treatment cream at night to begin training your skin to tolerate retinoic acids, as well as an antioxidant lotion or serum during the day. When you reach your forties, you'll be happy that you did.

## YOUR SKIN IN YOUR THIRTIES

Does life really shape the face that we have in our thirties? I think there's a lot of truth to that. We all have to face so many dilemmas and responsibilities when leaving our twenties. My father once told me that if I did not achieve my dreams and goals by the age of thirty, the chances were high that I probably never would. That literally made me panic. In the process, I earned a few worry lines. Later, at thirty-two, I successfully banished these lines with Botox, a small, relatively noninvasive, preventative step.

In our thirties, we are supposed to be living our dreams instead of making a living. This is the decade that we do most of our worrying and, inevitably, start to develop our frown lines and crow's feet. For most men and women, thirty is the key age when their career and personal goals are set in place. This is also when most people raise a family and have to juggle their parental obligations with a career. This is an even bigger task for women of the twenty-first century who struggle with the almost impossible combination of being a mother, a career woman, and a devoted wife. It is easy to see how our thirties leave a few impressions on our faces.

During this decade, cell turnover begins to slow down dramatically. The most noticeable consequences of this are dull skin and pigmentation changes. Because collagen and elastic fibers start to break down faster than they can be replenished, the skin starts to look tired and loses its radiance. The wrinkles of facial expressions are now visible even when we are not frowning or smiling. The dreaded "number 11" grooves between the brows begin to get deeper. This is usually more pronounced in patients who worry a great deal (hence the term worry lines). I've also seen it in a near-sighted writer who was habitually squinting at her computer screen. The thirties is the time to consider using Botox or Dysport® (onabotulinumtoxinA) to prevent the formation of facial expression lines that cause us to look angry, sad, or worried.

This decade is when your lifetime of sun damage begins to leave its mark. Brown spots start to show up around the sides of the face, and tiny red blood vessels begin to form around your nose and cheeks. When you have brown and red discoloration on your skin, these are considered competing chromophores. Instead of being reflected, red and brown spots compete to absorb light, leading to a sallow, tired looking skin. A skin that reflects light not only looks brighter, but the way the light reflects also makes small flaws on the skin almost undetectable—like a natural Photoshop touchup. So if skin has a lot of brown or red dyspigmentation, for instance, it will appear more wrinkled than it formerly did and pores will appear larger and more pronounced, even if they haven't changed size.

Due to a marked decrease in oil production between the twenties and the thirties, the skin starts to feel dry and crepe like. Moisturizing is a necessity, so if you used to get away without it, this is the time that you should start. I recommend two products, Make Me Younger™ (by Shino Bay Cosmetic Solutions) or Neutrogena® Positively Radiant, which both have subtle light-reflecting properties that make skin seem more luminous. However, avoid using heavy night creams because they can contribute to acne. At night instead use Spotlight or Be Sensitive Moisturizer by Shino Bay.

Other tips to help maintain a thirty-something skin are exfoliate the skin with a mild facial scrub, such as St. Ives® Apricot Scrub, once a week and to start using a facial cleansing brush, such as the Clarisonic®, the Olay® ProX, or the Neutrogena Wave Sonic, daily.

This is the age when I stress the use of a retinoic acid to prevent the breakdown of sun-damaged collagen and elastic fibers and increase the amount of new ones being produced. It's important at this age to build and maintain collagen and elastic fibers in order to prevent the thinning and sagging of the skin that typically occur during menopause.

## HOW TO PREPARE YOUR FACE FOR MENOPAUSE

1. Protect your skin from unnecessary sun exposure by using sunscreen daily.
2. Protect skin cells from free radicals by using an antioxidant serum or moisturizer.
3. Use a retinoic acid derivative, like tretinoin cream or retinol, at night.
4. Drink plenty of water and rest at night.
5. Give your skin a reason to rejuvenate by regularly doing treatments that stimulate collagen growth, such as microneedling, photofacials, chemical peels, and so on.

Often, men in their thirties worry about hair loss and receding hairlines. Thank God for men in the public eye who have made shaved heads a fashion statement, men like actors Vin Diesel, Bruce Willis, and Dwayne "the Rock" Johnson, musician and actor LL Cool J, rapper Pitbull, tennis player Andre Agassi, and male model Tyson Beckford. If you are balding or shave your head, remember that the skin on your scalp is sensitive. Apply sunscreen to this area every day and use an oil-based moisturizer.

## YOUR SKIN IN YOUR FORTIES

Our forties have never looked so good! This is an opinion shared by many in the beauty industry, who are excited about the plethora of devices and cosmeceuticals that are currently available to us. The forties are also a special decade because you still look young and feel young, but you have more wisdom than you did when you were younger. Most people like their lives more when they're in their forties because they know who they are and what they're doing. By your forties, unless you've been hiding under a rock, you've grown intellectually and emotionally, and this makes you an incredibly attractive person. People are attractive when they are in their prime.

During our forties, we come to appreciate the things that we probably took for granted in our younger years. This is considered the age of the emerging of wisdom and self-actualization, and our newfound confidence makes us all the more attractive to others. There is nothing sexier than a forty-something woman who still looks amazing. Many younger men today share this view. It is perhaps the reason why we have a proliferation of beautiful cougars here in Miami.

The same is true for men. Men in their forties who are well-kept, those who are fit and eat well, and who know themselves and their values, have a kind of mature confidence that is enormously attractive. Because men generally have thicker skin than women, and because of the fact that the micro-damage of daily shaving actually causes the skin to renew itself, until they hit their forties most men can get away simply with washing their faces with soap and water. They often don't even need moisturizer. At forty, men should begin using eye cream and face cream, as well as putting lotion on the rest of their bodies.

I see slogans everywhere stating: "The forties are the new twenties." There is a reason for that. Since we are living longer, we are no longer considered either mature or middle-aged in our forties. People in general are looking a lot younger at forty these days than a few decades ago. This is for two good reasons: First, we understand the aging face and skin a lot better than we used to. Second, we also have an enormous armamentarium of light-based treatments, fillers, neuromodulators like Botox or Dysport, and cosmeceuticals at our disposal to help people at forty look as if they are still in their thirties—or even their twenties.

I am one of those forty-somethings who still gets carded when I go out to bars or try to buy alcohol. Most of my patients think that I look like I am around twenty-five years of age. This doesn't bother me, because I do get the respect I deserve for my abilities. I honestly like myself better now in my forties than I ever have before.

Our era sounds good as long as you are a forty-something that looks younger. Unfortunately, our forties is also the decade when many of us start seeing telltale signs of aging. In this decade, every sign that emerged in our thirties will become even more accentuated.

Some characteristics of being in our forties are that our skin gets dry, has a rough texture, and appears dull. Areas of the skin with brown pigment increase in number and size, not only on the side of the face, but also in the center. Formerly tiny freckles may coalesce and become larger brown spots. Morning puffiness and swelling tend to take a while to dissipate, especially after having a fun night out drinking and eating salty food. The lines that began forming at thirty become deeper, and new lines join them to make the skin appear less smooth and resilient. The skin around the eyes continues to thin and begins to crinkle, especially in women.

The forties are when we start to lose our facial fat. As I often tell my patients, "This is when the fountain of youth starts to leave us." The face starts to descend due to the volume loss in the cheeks, and the skin, which is no longer able to compensate for the volume loss, begins to sag, as well. The corners of the mouth may turn down, making you look like you are frowning even when you are not. The lines from the corner of the nose to the corner of the mouth (nasolabial folds) also deepen.

In order to look amazing in this decade, one has to become diligent about replenishing what the body is losing. Using a retinoic acid and a rich moisturizer is recommended as a nighttime treatment. During the day, it is important to use an antioxidant serum or lotion, and to maintain adequate sun protection. Exfoliating once a week is also advisable to help the skin maintain its luster and smooth texture.

It is also important to replenish any volume loss. Otherwise, the skin will continue to descend and deflate. The constant pulling of gravity on the skin makes it stretch out and become inelastic, just like an old pair of underwear. Without restoration, everything will start to get wrinkled and drape around the mouth and jawline as you approach fifty. Thankfully, there are a plethora of fillers that can replenish the volume loss and keep the face in a younger position. If done correctly and in a timely manner, this can prevent the progression of the aging process.

Using Botox or Dysport neuromodulators to relax the muscles of facial expression not only freshens up the appearance, but these products can also discourage the formation of deep frown lines and crow's feet. In addition, there are a multitude of nonablative photofacials that work under the skin, promoting the formation of new collagen and elastic fibers to add to your skin's "bank account."

Supplements are also a good idea, especially for females. I always talk to my patients about menopause because it affects the bone and skin of a woman's body. My recommendations are to take a daily multivitamin containing vitamin D3, calcium, and vitamin C, and also take resveratrol supplements.

In their forties, men's body fat ratio starts increasing because their testosterone levels are dropping. They therefore should be more diligent about what they eat. My recommendation for men of this age is to take a daily multivitamin containing vitamin C, vitamin D3, saw palmetto, and omega-3s.

There are so many great things about being forty. We are relatively healthy, have accumulated important life lessons, are financially more stable than we were before we reached this age when we just entering in the prime of our careers, and we have a much better idea of what's good for us—and what's not. Although many people fear their forties when they're younger, because it's when changes really start happening to their bodies, most of us really enjoy arriving here. My recommendation is to embrace your age and do all you can to replenish whatever is starting to fade. In our forties we have the choice to feel young at heart as well as in mind, body, and spirit in the way that are predecessors did not.

## YOUR SKIN IN YOUR FIFTIES

I remember when being fifty meant being old. They used to call it being "over the hill," but they don't say that anymore. People at fifty today are looking younger and feeling sexier and more energetic than ever. The days of raising children are over, and a second wave of life has begun. Women are even lying less and less about their ages. My grandmother was forever forty-five until it became impossible to lie any more. Then she was forever fifty-five. These are not the same fifty-year-old women from the past. The fifties are the new thirties! Many of my patients are bragging about their ages—because being fifty and looking great is definitely something to brag about.

The secret of reaching fifty and looking and feeling fabulous involves being well-informed about the changes that are happening to our bodies as we age and taking the right steps to replenish the ground substances and elements that get depleted with age. We have to eat well-balanced meals, drink plenty of water, get uninterrupted sleep, and respond to stress in appropriate ways, find our joy, maintain our sense of humor, stay out of direct sunlight, and take care of our skin.

Sometimes during my consultations and seminars, I get too graphic about the changes that happen to an aging face. From the younger set, I will hear comments such as, "Oh, God, I had better kill myself now" and "Is this what I have to look forward to?" When this happens, I immediately explain that someone who is well informed can prevent many of these changes and maintain his or her youthful features longer. Also, bear in mind that if you love yourself only because of how you look, then perhaps your life could have more depth and heart and soul to it. The people to emulate as we continue to move through the decades of our lives are those who are constantly finding new and surprising ways to challenge themselves. These individuals remain youthful because they are exploring the world and its possibilities, and often reinventing themselves periodically. Their lesson for us is to choose to make the best of each decade of our lives.

Remember, men and women who prepare for aging by eating right, getting exercise, and avoiding cigarette smoke, and excessive sun exposure, always look younger than their actual chronological ages.

When we reach the fifth decade, the changes that we observed in earlier decades become more pronounced. This is especially true for women because of their more extreme hormonal fluctuations. Of course, male hormones also diminish after the thirties, causing accumulating belly fat, drier skin, loss of elasticity of the skin, brown spots, and baldness. The breakdown of collagen and elastic fibers that began in our thirties is now in full speed, causing a major sagging of the skin. The skin may also become thin and translucent, and many of the facial blood vessels may become more visible. All of the wrinkles around the forehead and eyes become deeper, and the vertical lip lines start to manifest. These lines are usually hereditary, but can also be caused by pursing the lips when talking or smoking.

This is a good opportunity for me to illustrate how a deficit of collagen and elastic fibers can cause the sagging and wrinkling of the skin. Have you ever wondered why men are not as prone to vertical lip lines as women? It's because most men shave. The act of shaving injures the skin daily. The skin responds to the shaving injury by generating new collagen and elastic fibers, resulting in the daily accumulation of connective tissues.

The brown spots that appeared decades earlier become greater both in number and in size when people are fifty. Some of these spots even acquire a texture similar to barnacles. The blood vessels become more pronounced and richer in color.

The fifties are also the time when the malposition of fat becomes more evident. The fat pads on the cheeks, temples, and around the mouth continue to disappear, causing the skin to sag even more than in your thirties and forties. In addition, fat accumulates under the eyes, chin, and jawline, causing added downward traction on the skin. In other words, with a little help from gravity, the face descends.

Until now, all of the volume loss on the face that we have been concerned about came from the loss of facial fat. Entering the fifth decade of life, there is evidence of volume loss not only from fat, but also from the bony elements of the face. This bone volume loss is more prominent in females due to the effects of menopause; however, it also happens to men. Men should take the same steps toward being healthy that women take so that you can avoid adverse impact from andropause.

Have you ever noticed that the most problematic area in

the aging of a woman is around her mouth? Women have the most changes from bone around the jaw. As you may recall from reading Chapter 2, we can expect some bone loss as time passes. Around age fifty, when the bone in the lower jaw starts to decrease in mass, the soft tissues reposition, causing wrinkling around the lips and eventually severe sagging in the mouth. The bone above the mouth also loses mass, undermining the support of the midface.

For this reason, I ensure that my female patients who are serious about facial age prevention supplement their diets with calcium and vitamin D3 and take a bone density test to check for osteopenia and osteoporosis. As women age, their bones tend to become more porous and prone to fractures. This reduction in bone mass is due to depletion of calcium and protein. If you have any bone loss or brittleness, nowadays it can be treated. Medication and bioidentical hormone supplements are showing promising results in the prevention of bone loss.

The loss of volume of fat from the cheeks leads to the sagging of the lower eyelid and the formation of "bags" under the eyes (see the discussion in Chapter 1).

All of my patients at age fifty are advised to use some form of retinoic acid, a heavy cream moisturizer at night for the face and eyes, an antioxidant formulation—either a serum or a moisturizer—and a physical sunblock during the day. Once or twice a year, I recommend undergoing photofacials with lasers that have the capability to destroy old collagen and elastic fibers and replace them with new ones. How often depends on the laser technology that is chosen. If needed, I may also use lasers that cause tissue tightening to prevent the descent and deflation of the face. Be sure to discuss this option with your skin care specialist as soon as you start seeing or feeling structural changes on your skin—change of position, changes in tone and elasticity. This type of treatment helps the skin accommodate facial fat volume loss. Laser treatments can help eliminate the brown spots and facial veins that cause the skin to look sallow and tired. We'll discuss different laser treatments in depth in Chapter 9.

One simple test of your skin's resilience is the snap test. If you pull on the skin with a little pinch, it should bounce back into place immediately. If it takes longer to go back to position—which granted will sometimes happen if you are dehydrated, too—then the skin's collagen and elastic fibers are likely getting lower.

More and more people are taking advantage of technological advances and paying attention to their facial fat volume loss, including wondering how much collagen and elastic fibers are in their facial "bank accounts." They are finding that plastic surgery intervention does not have to be in their future plans, as their faces are still in generally the same position as they were decades before. Reaching age fifty is truly a blessing. As technology and research continue to bring more and more life extenders, being fifty today also means looking and feeling better and better.

## YOUR SKIN IN YOUR SIXTIES

Joan Rivers once said, "Looking fifty is great . . . if you are sixty!" If there is anyone who knows a lot about not wanting to look her age, it's Ms. Rivers. I don't care what anyone else says, I love her! She has undergone numerous transformations in one lifetime. Perhaps because we know a lot more about volume depletion, her look these days is softer and more natural than it was in previous decades.

I have been meeting many beautiful ladies in their sixties who are not only gorgeous but have also managed to dodge some of the effects of time. My stepmother, Frances, is one of them. She has never had any plastic surgery, her skin is flawless and lineless, and her volume is impeccable. All it took was the help of my lasers, a syringe, and some artistry. Frances has always taken really good preventative care of her skin, and she also hops on a flight from Los Angeles to Fort Lauderdale at the first hint of an issue so I can treat her before matters go too far.

Another amazing sixty-something woman is the actress Suzanne Somers. This ageless beauty really understands how to maintain her youth and vitality from the inside out. She is living proof of the benefits of always replenishing what our bodies can no longer produce or assimilate. From her healthy eating habits to her enthusiasm about bioidentical hormones, Suzanne Somers has inspired many women and men of all ages to be proactive about looking younger.

When men reach their sixties, the advantages they've had with their skin and bones disappear due to the hormonal shifts they undergo. Mother Nature levels the playing field, and men may even start developing osteoporosis. Therefore, the same advice I give women should govern the behavior of both genders from this stage onward.

Changes that affect the skin in earlier decades, including volume loss, continue. The skin gets thinner and blotchy. The brown spots continue to get darker and coalesce into larger ones. The blood vessels on the face seem larger and purplish, like little rivers on a map. The light absorption from these colorful lesions causes the skin to further lose its luster.

As the skin continues to break down more collagen and elastic fibers than it can create, wrinkles, creases, and frown lines become ever more pronounced. In addition, as gravity continues to pull on this less elastic skin, it further sags and elongates. This is why excess skin sometimes needs to be removed during a facelift or an eye lift.

Fat malposition is an increasingly big problem in this decade. In addition to the facial fat loss and concomitant loss of facial fullness we've already spoken about and see in our fifties, the fat pockets around the jawline, eyes, and under the chin become discernible as separate entities, disrupting the defining arcs and convexities of a once-youthful face. The changes to the bony elements of the face continue occurring and become more profound. These lead to decreased support for the midface, as additional negative downward vectors are added to the same face that has been descending for decades. Now we can easily see the so-called triangle of youth in the process of becoming the pyramid of old age.

During this decade, heavy moisturizing creams are recommended to maintain the hydration of the skin. Moisturizers containing soy can help diminish the production of brown spots. Using sunblock and antioxidants to protect the skin during the day is also recommended. At night, it is advisable to use a cream, lotion, or serum containing retinoic acid to increase the amount of collagen and elastic fibers in the skin. Moisturizing agents that contain hyaluronic acid will help your skin appear plumper and suppler. Drinking plenty of water, taking a multivitamin and vitamin D3, resveratrol, and calcium supplements is part of my daily recommendation for healthy skin at this age. It's incredibly important to stay active with a good fitness program that includes some cardiovascular exercise and some strength building exercise. If you become sedentary you're in trouble.

When combined with lasers that tighten the skin, photofacials create collagen and elastic fibers. These treatments, which use exposure to laser light, can improve the tone and texture of the skin. Replenishing volume loss with fillers may not only improve the overall appearance of the face, but possibly also help to halt the aging process on the face.

In individuals for whom it is already too late to correct the effects of volume loss and inelastic skin, plastic surgery is an option. However, after the surgery, the volume loss, and skin changes do need to be corrected. If the volume and the quality of the skin are not addressed, the patient will look like a person who has had plastic surgery without the benefit of looking any younger—same age with a tighter face.

## YOUR SKIN IN YOUR SEVENTIES
## AND BEYOND

I have always wondered how old someone has to be to stop caring about his or her looks. I live in South Florida where many people come to retire and live a life of leisure. Most of these retirees play golf and tennis, swim, and lead busy social lives; so looking good is a must for them. They usually tell me, "I don't need to look like I'm thirty—I just don't want to look tired and saggy."

The truth is that we really never stop caring about the way we look. The other day one of my seventy-plus patients told me, "We don't stop caring about what we look like, but sometimes our priorities change." Wise words. When you are dealing with a serious illness, for example, worrying about your looks could seem rather insignificant or even inappropriate.

In the past, before all of the new technological advances that are described in this book, we had nothing to do but accept with grace that we were going to age and it would take its toll on our faces. It happened to our parents and to our parents' parents, and to their ancestors. After all, aging is a natural part of life. However, people did not formerly have the life spans that we have now. We are living longer, and it doesn't make sense to ignore the fact that we now have the resources to improve our appearances and halt the "darn clock."

We all want to be able to match how we feel on the inside with how we look. I have many patients over the age of seventy who look and feel amazing. I always refer to my beautiful patient, Joan, who is over seventy and still looks beautiful and leads an active lifestyle. She takes care of her garden, exercises, and has the figure of a yoga or a Pilates instructor. As a result of her genes and health and fitness regimen, she has an unbelievable peaches-and-cream skin that is smooth, thick, and flawless. She is a role model for her younger friends, showing how well someone can age when she takes the right steps to replenish and restore what the process of aging takes away.

With all of these new advances in technology, everyone can improve their health and vitality and have beautiful skin at any age. All it takes is knowledge of how the aging process works and being willing to take the right steps toward restoration. Studies have shown that people who take care of themselves through-out their lives not only look and feel great, but are also healthier.

The decades beyond the seventies bring a lot more of the same. The skin continues to sag and wrinkle. The dark spots become larger and thicker. The veins on the face get larger in size and number. The wrinkles from previous decades continue to get deeper and deeper. The volume loss from fat and bone continues, causing the facial skin to collapse around the mouth and change the ratios and proportions of what once was a younger face.

The skin during these decades tend to be thinner and drier, so I recommend using a heavy moisturizer and continuing with a retinoic acid at nighttime to nourish and repair the skin cells and to replenish the reserve of collagen and elastic fibers.

During the day, continue sun protection with a physical sun-block and an antioxidant serum. Using a heavy moisturizer in the morning may also be required if the skin is still lacking proper hydration. By using a serum containing hyaluronic acid to draw water to the skin and then layering a heavy moisturizer on top of that to occlude it, you can prevent water loss and improve the texture and suppleness of the skin.

Using lasers to tighten the skin and crank up the production of new collagen and elastic fibers is also extremely helpful. The lasers that I use for this age group are safe, efficient, and require very little downtime or discomfort during recovery.

Members of this age group, as well as earlier age groups, benefit from restoring the ongoing volume depletion that occurs with age. It is amazing to see the youthful appearances of patients who maintain an adequate amount of volume on their faces. They sometimes seem twenty years younger than their chronological ages! I have learned a great deal about the aging process by studying the faces of my good-looking older patients to see what they have in common. They all have facial fat, amazing cheekbones, and a longer internal clock than most people. Because they have been genetically blessed I tell them they should thank their moms and dads for such a gift.

Eleanor Roosevelt once said, "Beautiful young people are accidents of nature, but beautiful old people are works of art." So honor yourself by making an effort to maintain your skin and facial volume no matter your age. Rest assured that you can get results if you put in the effort.

CHAPTER 7

# "Botox Saved My Marriage"

When I opened Shino Bay Cosmetic Dermatology and Laser Institute, a good friend of mine gave me a small pillow that read, "Botox saved my marriage." I could not help laughing when I saw it, but later I began to wonder . . . *Has Botox* really *saved some people's marriages?* I imagined a marriage in which a husband could never tell if his wife was mad at him because she always wore the same happy expression on her face. His life would be absolutely blissful, right?

All kidding aside, the truth is that anything is possible. One report found Botox® to be useful in helping people with depression. The study, conducted by Eric Finzi, M.D., Ph.D., and Erica Wasserman, Ph.D., published in the May 2006 issue of *Journal of Dermatologic Surgery,* found that after having Botox injected into their forehead furrows, nine out of ten women had a significant reduction in their symptoms. Although other experts may disagree with the results of this pilot study, many patients report a big improvement in their moods following their injections.

My patients frequently tell me how happy they feel once they've had their Botox.

As a college student at UCLA, I had first-hand experience with the relationship between muscle relaxation and mental health. I was extremely stressed, and though not to the point of being depressed, I was so anxious that I felt that my upper teeth might come loose from all the tooth grinding and jaw clenching I was doing. Of course, the very thought of this stressed me out even more! I went to get some counseling on campus and found a counselor who shared a trick with me.

Whenever I felt myself getting stressed, she told me to fake a smile and pay attention to how my body reacted. I thought she was insane, but I had nothing to lose. I tried it and—*voila*—it worked! My body quickly started to relax and feel good. The moment I started to smile, I could feel my back and shoulder muscles relax. Along with some other relaxation techniques that I incorporated into my lifestyle, I was soon able to get rid of my stress on command.

There is a direct connection between the muscles used for facial expressions and the brain. If I was able to alleviate my stress by faking a smile, then maybe it was possible to help alleviate depression by preventing the muscles that cause a face to look sad or angry from working. We are well aware that there are gestures and movements that arise with our emotions. The more you do those movements and gestures, the more amplified those emotions become. This feedback mechanism operates between the brain and the muscles to express emotions. Therefore, if Botox can prevent someone from frowning, it should also alleviate or lessen the intensity of the depressed emotion.

Botox® Cosmetic is a trademarked name for onabotulinumtoxinA. Considered a *neuromodulator,* it was first approved to soften the lines formed between the eyebrows and more recently for the treatment of the wrinkles by the outer corner of the eyes known as crow's feet. Its wrinkle-erasing properties were discovered when eye doctors noticed that patients who were treated with Botox for muscular problems looked refreshed and wrinkle free afterward. Originally dermatological use was an "off-label" treatment. Now such use is an "on-label" treatment. The aesthetic effects of Botox are rewarding, and the results can last anywhere from three to six months.

Although Botox is a wonderful drug, I believe that it's possible to have too much of a good thing. If a little Botox can save someone's marriage by keeping a spouse happy, remember that too much could really make things go south. During my consultations, I explain that I am a minimalist with respect to my Botox administration and technique. Aesthetically, I believe less is more. I want my patients to look younger and refreshed, but that the work should be 100 percent undetectable. If people can tell a mile away that you have been "Botoxed," then it defeats the purpose.

Facial expressions are very important in the human experience. We are wired to instinctively respond to other people's facial expressions. If you smile at people, they in turn will usually smile back. There are verbal and nonverbal aspects to communication. If you only have one expression for all your emotions, this will not only make you look inappropriate and bizarre, but it also may cause social isolation and discord.

Studies have shown that when spouses argue it is often because they are not correctly reading each other's facial expressions. Miscommunication can be treacherous and devastating in a relationship. Therefore, if a husband cannot correctly read his wife's nonverbal expressions because she has been over treated with Botox and Dysport, then Botox could potentially become a culprit in the demise of their marriage.

We have fifty-three muscles that we use to create the 7,000 or so facial expressions we use to convey our emotions. It's important that we can look at someone's face and get a proper reading about what they are attempting to indicate. If what is said verbally does not correspond with the facial expression, we may be apprehensive about accepting the information that has been given to us. There's an implication of sarcasm or lying. Imagine if you dumped a beer on someone's shirt and said, "Sorry," but had a slight smirk on your face. It could lead to an altercation.

This is why some news reporters and actors are not allowed to use Botox while they are under contract to their stations. Just imagine a television reporter relaying the news of a horrible accident with a face incapable of showing any sympathy. As you can see, facial feedback is very important! Even in the world of texting and emailing, we often send a smiley face icon or a sad face icon to let people know what kind of mood we are in.

Botox is not for everyone. With certain facial anatomies, it can make some people look bizarre. People with high brow arches, for example, may look perpetually surprised. I like to call this the Jack Nicholson look. The injection technique often needs to be modified accordingly to gender, age, and anatomy in order to make Botox work for the benefit of the patient. I see too many people walking around with frozen faces or that perpetually astonished look. It is uncomfortable to have conversations with them because there is no feedback mechanism in faces with such little movement.

I tell my patients who are either in a sales-oriented job or single and dating to beware of getting too much Botox in order to avoid the risk of being incorrectly perceived as dishonest or uninterested. Another consequence of being over "Botoxed" is that the inactive muscles lose their tone and then people's foreheads start to look longer. Sometimes, the head of the eyebrows descend and collapse towards the bridge of the nose.

When over-Botoxed people come to my office, they usually say, "Botox used to lift my brows like this (holding their brows up with their fingers), and now I can't get them up! What can I do?" The solution is to get an endoscopic brow lift.

I have noticed that when people cannot move their foreheads at all, they start to compensate by moving the tiny little muscles on their nose, causing them to form bunny lines, or what I like to call a Klingon's nose. A good solution is to use tiny amounts of Botox on the nose area to discourage the formation of these nose lines.

I love Botox. It's one of the most gratifying procedures I do in my practice in terms of results in the appearance and self-esteem. It is minimally invasive and can really turn the clock back a few years—and maintain youthfulness that way. However, it needs to be done correctly. The amount used should be enough to relax the muscle, but there should be enough muscle tone remaining to have some degree of movement on the face.

I have met many potential clients who are so afraid of the aging process that they obsess about it. They do not want to move a facial muscle one bit. I usually advise them to seek the services of other physicians who are comfortable doing a more intensive type of injection technique. My patients are the ambassadors of my practice and a reflection of my work. It is important to me that they look as natural as possible.

Like any other medication, there may be complications or adverse reactions to Botox. At the amount used for cosmetics, the adverse reactions are minimal. There have been a lot of reports in the media about Botox being dangerous; however, most of the serious adverse reactions to the drug that have been reported occurred with patients with cerebral palsy or paraplegics, whose conditions required a thousand times more units than are used for cosmetic purposes. Of course, the likelihood of a serious adverse reaction increases commensurate with the quantity of the drug that is used.

I remember being a resident when a friend of mine who was a nurse called to let me know that four people were severely ill from Botox. I panicked because three days earlier I had treated her, myself, and four other friends. Afraid that we might have gotten a bad batch, I quickly called Allergan, the manufacturer, to get some information. They reassured me that the Botox that had caused this incident was not from them. Later, it was discovered that some doctors from Florida had been using a form of botulinumtoxinBTX that had been manufactured for animal research. It was highly concentrated and extremely cheap to purchase.

This is an example of greed at its worst! They could use very little of the BTX, dilute it with tons of saline solution, and charge the same amount of money as doctors who were using the real deal. The profit would have been astronomical if it were not for the divine law of karma. It turns out that the doctor using the fake Botox had injected himself and three of his friends. I know that all of them went through hell and back during this ordeal, and I am happy to report that they are all doing well now.

After that dreaded incident, the media, as usual, took the news and ran with it. Many people became afraid of using Botox. Although I firmly believe that in the right hands—and in the small quantities that are used for aesthetic purposes—Botox is extremely safe, patients should be aware of all potential side effects and drug interactions before receiving Botox treatment. In addition, if a patient has any disease that causes the muscles to weaken, such as amyotrophic lateral sclerosis (Lou Gehrig's disease) or myasthenia gravis, or has problems with swallowing, breathing, or any motor neuropathic disease, then onabotulinumtoxinA is an absolute contraindication and should not be used. There has not been a confirmed severe adverse reaction to date when Botox has been utilized for cosmetic reasons or for hyperhidrosis. The most common side effect that I have seen in a few of my patients (including myself) is a mild to moderate, short-lasting headache that can usually be alleviated with Tylenol®.

The Botox brand dominated the cosmetic market for years, and until recently, it was the only onabotulinumtoxinA administered in the United States. In July 2009, the FDA approved Dysport, a new type of onabotulinumtoxinA that, according to its makers, is supposed to act faster and last longer than Botox. I have used Botox for so many years that I am comfortable and proficient with it; however, many of my patients have started to request the new drug. Since I began also using Dysport, I have noticed that it works better in certain areas with less amount of the product. I love, for example, the way the eye area responds to this new product. If patients have strong muscles between their brows, Dysport is a good choice, as well. Since then, a new type of neuromodulator has arrived in the aesthetic market: Xeomin® (incobotulinumtoxinA).   This new neuromodulator has the same mode of onset and duration as Botox, according to Merz, its maker.

Whether I am using Botox or Dysport, one thing is certain: None of my patients will leave my clinic with a generic, motionless face.

# CHAPTER 8

# Fill Me Up

ermal fillers have become an important breakthrough in treating the effects of aging. They can be used to eliminate dermal creases and wrinkles, raise depressed scars, augment lips, and replenish soft tissue volume loss. We have certainly come a long way from the use of collagen, which had a high incidence of allergic reactions and a relatively short duration (about three months). Recently, a plethora of new fillers have eliminated the need for allergy testing and boast increased durability.

I use injectable dermal fillers in my practice to prevent the advancement of facial aging and to ensure that my patients do not become premature candidates for surgical intervention. As I mentioned at the beginning of this book, the volumetric properties of facial fat make it a key ingredient of the fountain of youth. It is becoming widely accepted among dermatologists and plastic surgeons that volume depletion, due to facial fat loss and bone loss, is responsible for the vast majority of changes in the aging face.

It really bothers me when prospective patients come into my office with deflated faces and fillers in their nasolabial folds. I explain that using a filler to eliminate their creases without lifting and reshaping their cheeks only increases the number of negative vectors on the face, thereby accelerating the aging process. It's Physics 101. The downward force from the weight of the filler together with the effect of gravity causes the skin to become less elastic and begin to sag, especially around the eyes.

Most people start to lose their volume from fat and soft tissue around age forty. I have, however, also met some genetically blessed individuals in their fifties and sixties who still have most of the fat cells in their faces. They look at least twenty years younger than their chronological ages.

Around the fifth decade, we also start to suffer volume depletion from bone remodeling. This type of change is more pronounced in women due to menopause. Women tend to lose more bone mass in the jawbones than men, as well as more soft tissue in the upper face. As skeletal volume is lost, the soft tissues collapse around the mouth and the skin wrinkles. I often see women in their fifties who still have perfect skin in their upper faces and yet have severe wrinkles and loose skin around their mouths.

In addition, we can all see what happens to the cheeks of someone relatively young who has poor dentition. Due to the condition of the teeth, their faces appear sunken in, which causes the face to look old because the skin has become wrinkled and saggy. It is especially important for women who care about slowing down the clock to supplement their diets with calcium, magnesium, and vitamin D3. Taking good personal care of their teeth, minimizing grinding at night, and having regular visits to the dentist should be part of their age-prevention routines.

Now that we've discerned that volume in the face is a key ingredient of the fountain of youth, we've found that rebuilding volume loss is an easy and effective way to rejuvenate an aging face. Like everything else, however, some people take it to the extreme. I have seen many people on the streets, including celebrities, with overfilled cheeks that make them look like cartoon characters from a galaxy far, far away. My heart sinks when they come into my office looking like that. I wonder, *Do they see what I see?*

Volume restoration should be undetectable! In my opinion, if someone looks filled from a mile away, it's a catastrophe! I remember going through the pages of *InTouch* magazine at the airport and seeing a picture of Lisa Rinna from the original *Melrose Place*. Her cheeks were so freakishly inflated that I could not see her beautiful face. Unfortunately, there are many other women walking around who look just like that. It's almost as if the Cabbage Patch Kids have grown up and are making a comeback as life-sized adult dolls.

When it comes to fillers, more is not necessarily better. As we can all agree, there is such a thing as too much filler. In my consultations, I stress my philosophy that less is more. I can always add more filler if required, but I cannot take it out. It's a misconception that more filler is going to slow down the darn clock. If anything, getting too much filler will speed it up even faster.

Here's an analogy that explains why this is so. When plastic surgeons need to do breast reconstructions, they sometimes need extra skin to recreate the breast. So, what do they do? They use tissue expanders that stretch the skin in order to have enough material to create a breast. This illustrates the potential outcome of having overfilled cheeks for a long time: the skin becomes stretched to the point of no return. Should this happen, the only way to keep those cheeks up is to inflate them with more filling product, leaving the person they belong to looking even more bizarre. If they should come to their senses and decide not to have that look again, the skin will be so stretched out that they will have to assume the look of da-da da-da daaaaa Underdog! Unfortunately, surgery may be required in order to correct this look.

I've had many such patients with overfilled cheeks who came to me for a more natural look. I was surprised and intrigued upon examining their skin. It was translucent, much like a balloon, and it was spongy, like Stretch Armstrong, an action figure doll from the 1970s. After waiting for the product in their cheeks to deflate, I used a collagen-stimulating filler to thicken the skin and rebuild their volume to a more natural and refreshed look.

Injectable fillers are taking center stage in the world of aesthetics. They are helping to solve some of the major issues of facial aging: reshaping of the face, enhancing facial contours, and correcting asymmetries. Every year, new fillers with clever and alluring names are added to the already substantial list of FDA-approved injectable fillers, creating a lot of confusion for patients trying to select the ideal filler for their particular needs. In this next section, I will discuss the most popular injectable fillers, as well as the ones that I use most frequently in my practice. My intention is for it to serve as a veritable insider's guide to injectable fillers.

## SILICONE

Silicon is the most abundant nonmetallic element, next to oxygen, that exists in the Earth's crust. Although it does not occur in a free elemental state, it is found almost everywhere in the form of silicon dioxide (silica) and complex silicates. It is typically found in nature in sand, quartz, brackish water, and the ocean.

Silicones are synthetic polymers called polydimethylsiloxanes (PDMS) that are made by combining oxygen and silicon under high temperature and pressure. According to the amount of cross linking, silicones can exist as solids, liquids, or gels. The silicone fluids are made from linear chains of PDMS. These fluid silicones exist in a variety of grades according to the level of impurities that they contain. Industrial silicone tends to have a large amount of impurities and is used to make lubricants, varnishes, and binders. In cosmetics, it is used in lotions and potions for hair and skin.

Liquid silicones are not approved to inject into the body for cosmetic applications. The only FDA-approved use for liquid silicones is in the case of retinal detachment, where it is injected into the eyes to prevent blindness.

However, liquid silicones can be used "off label" to treat certain maladies. The use of off-label medications and medical devices was sanctioned by the 1997 Amendment to the Federal Food, Drug, and Cosmetic Act 6, which states that a physician can legally use, off label, any medication or device that has been approved for other purposes provided that the doctor believes that it can effectively treat or cure a patient's complaint. In the hands of an experienced physician, silicone makes a great permanent filler. However, it has acquired a bad reputation due to the injections of nonmedical grade silicone by non-physicians.

The microdroplet technique is the safest and most predictable approach for injecting this product. The most commonly used silicon-based products in the United States are Silikon® 1000 and AdatoSil® 5000. These are FDA-approved, purified, medical-grade silicones used for postoperative retinal tamponade during vitreoretinal surgery. For the last thirty years, however, it has also been used off label as dermal filler by plastic surgeons and dermatologists. In fact, it was the first injectable filler ever used around the world.

The injection of silicone oil into the skin triggers a foreign body response and low-grade inflammation. Since silicone is an inert substance and cannot be broken down by the body, the body has to do something to prevent chronic inflammation or the rejection of this foreign substance from occurring. The almighty and savvy human body does something miraculous: It tells the fibroblast cells in the skin to produce collagen around the product to wall it off and encapsulate it. This process continues until the body recognizes the collagen-encapsulated silicone droplet as itself and stops the low-grade inflammatory response. It's similar to the process by which pearls are formed. Pearls are the result of a biological process in which an oyster tries to protect itself from foreign substances and irritants, such as sand (which is made from silica), organic material, and parasites.

Understanding the foreign body reaction is a great way to illustrate what can go wrong if silicone of a nonpurified medical grade is used in a cosmetic procedure. The more impurities the silicone has, the higher the potential for it to cause chronic inflammation and large granuloma formations. This happened to the beautiful Priscilla Presley when she allowed a non-licensed physician to inject industrial, low-grade silicone (the kind used to lubricate auto parts) in her face. Besides the obvious cosmetic consequences, it also created a permanent medical condition. I am just thankful that she did not incur a more serious consequence, such as losing her life. She is and will always be a beautiful woman in my eyes.

In my practice, I have seen many victims of botched injections at the hands of improperly trained physicians or non-physicians. Unfortunately, there is nothing I can do other than to reduce the size of the nodules and provide comfort from pain or inflammation. (Note: some individuals can form granulomas years after being injected even with medical-grade silicone. We do not yet understand why this occurs.)

In my practice, I use Silikon 1000 to correct small defects or depressions on the skin (perhaps caused by trauma or acne scars) that are too deep to respond to laser treatments. After six to nine weeks, I can add more of the product. I am not comfortable using silicone to augment areas that need a large volume. If the body decides to reject the product, I can't just punch it out the same way I could if it were injected into a very small area without leaving a large defect.

Purified medical-grade silicone has a very small incidence of allergic reactions. Nevertheless, I would hate to encounter a case of a reaction with a product that is permanent. Since the face constantly changes throughout the decades, I don't like to use permanent fillers that remain in place while the rest of the face ages and drops around them. This can be deforming. In addition, once patients have had silicone injected into their faces or lips, it limits the number of other injectable fillers that can be safely used in those areas.

## FAT TRANSFER

Fat transfer is a two-part procedure in which fat is withdrawn from a patient's donor site with a syringe or with a liposuction cannula. The donor site for the harvesting of fat is usually the abdomen, hips, or buttocks. The harvested fat is prepared by clearing away all the blood and plasma according to the physician's preferred method. Once the fat is ready to be transferred, the patient is prepped and cleansed to reduce the risk of infections, and the fat is injected into the areas to be enhanced or corrected. Since the fat comes right from the patient's body, there is no reason to worry about allergic reactions.

Depending on the type of procedure and the surgeon, fat can be injected in small amounts over a period of time or in large volumes all at once. Injecting small amounts of fat causes less trauma to the treatment area. Although this means that less downtime is needed for recovery, multiple treatments become necessary. The fat is usually stored in freezers to be used for subsequent treatments. When using the large-volume technique, there is more swelling, bruising, and downtime. The increase in trauma to the donor site can necessitate the application of compression bandages for a week or more.

The durability of the fat transfer depends on the technique used, the amount of volume injected, and the patient's unique individual ability to metabolize fat. Physicians and other researchers have observed that fat transfer can last anywhere from six months to seven years.

While observing fat transfer techniques during my residency, I found them messy, unpredictable, and a bit barbaric. Although I was never attracted to this procedure, many of my colleagues love it and get amazing results. I prefer to use fillers that are not permanent—because in my opinion permanent fillers can lead to permanent problems.

In addition, I have met individuals who originally looked great after having a fat transfer. Then, as they started to lose bone mass underneath the filler, they looked a bit inappropriate. There's nothing worse than to have the fat volume of a twenty-year old superimposed on an aged-looking skull. Patients that come to me in this condition are difficult to treat because they have too much volume from fat grafting. It is impossible for me to take measures to imitate the appearance of bone volume without making the problem look worse.

## COLLAGENS

In Chapter 3, we discussed how collagen is the main protein that provides structural support for the skin and the connective tissues. Collagen and elastic fibers are woven like threads to form a structural framework that is responsible for the smooth and supple appearance of youthful skin, as well as the healthy growth of cells and blood vessels.

In the early 1970s, researchers from Stanford University were successful in extracting a purified form of bovine collagen that was derived from cows. In 1976, this form of collagen was ready to be used in patients. From then until 2002, bovine collagen was the only available filler approved by the FDA for cosmetic use in patients in the United States. Although patients were happy with the results, in only three months or less the nice corrections were pretty much gone. Additionally, since this type of collagen came from cows, allergy tests were required. Although some allergy test results appeared normal for a week or two, allergic reactions would sometimes show up later, leaving many patients wishing for safer, longer-lasting filler.

Zyderm® and Zyplast® (made by Allergan) were the first bovine-derived collagen products to appear on the market (in 1981 and 1985, respectively). They were routinely used to improve na-solabial folds and to augment lips. The main difference between the Zyderm and Zyplast formulations was durability. Zyplast was more crosslinked, causing it to be thicker and more resistant to degradation. Unfortunately, studies showed that about 3 percent of patients were allergic to them. Many people were left wondering whether the investment was worth it.

In their quest to create the perfect collagen filler that would eliminate the incidence of allergic reactions, researchers found a way to generate human-derived filler. This may sound a bit crazy, but Cosmoderm® and Cosmoplast® synthesized their collagens from cells originally extracted from human baby foreskin.

Cosmoderm and Cosmoplast were both FDA approved in March 2003. Cosmoderm is a soft, malleable product that is perfect for fine lines and to outline the upper lip. Cosmoplast, which is crosslinked and thicker, is well suited for the body of the lip and to inject into the nasolabial folds. Since Cosmoderm and Cosmoplast do not require skin testing, they became the first same-day, single-visit collagen fillers approved in the United States. (Note: patients with a history of serious allergic reactions or known allergies to lidocaine should not use these products.) These fillers have a similar durability to Zyderm and Zyplast. The need for a longer lasting collagen-derived product was not met until 2008.

Evolence® became the new kid on the block in the world of injectable collagen fillers in 2008. It was introduced to the United States after it had been used in Canada, Europe, Asia, and Israel for several years. Evolence has an impeccable safety profile. It is a collagen-derived filler that does not require a skin allergy test. It does not come from a human source, but from kosher pigs from Israel. *Oy vay!* As you may or may not know, there are many genetic similarities between pigs and humans. This is why surgeons have been using pig valves for heart valve replacement surgery for the last twenty years. Many of the pig's proteins are close in sequence and structure to human proteins.

Although porcine collagen does not require a skin allergy test, patients with a history of severe allergies or anaphylaxis should not use this product.

Collagen is rarely used as filler in the United States anymore because hyaluronic acid is a method that is much preferred. So although it can work, it is no longer the best option.

## HYALURONIC ACIDS

When we think about acids, we usually think about caustic solutions that cause chemical burns when improperly handled. Hyaluronic acids, however, are not caustic. They are simply naturally occurring polysaccharides—natural sugars—that are found in every tissue of the body. These are necessary to promote the creation and movement of new cells. They are also an essential component in cell-to-cell interactions, growth, metabolism, and nutrition. Hyaluronic acids are highly concentrated in the skin, vitreous humor of the eyes, and in the cartilage. They are a primary component of synovial fluid, which serves as a lubricant in the joints. Basically, hyaluronic acids serve to lubricate, nurture, and cushion the body.

In the skin, they are found between the collagen and elastic fibers. One of their main functions is to deliver nutrition and hydration to the skin's cells. Over 50 percent of the body's hyaluronic acids are found in the skin (7–8 grams per average adult human). They give the skin its volume, turgor, and pliability. Their unique ability to bind to water up to a thousand times their volume in the skin has made them a popular ingredient in skin care products and as injectable filler. This property allows them to fill and correct every nook and cranny of an aging skin.

Hyaluronic acids are derived from animal and bacterial sources. In my practice, I use brands of viscoelastic, bacteria-derived hyaluronic acids, such as Restylane® (made by Galderma), Perlane® (made by Galderma), Juvéderm® Ultra and Juvéderm

Ultra Plus (made by Allergan), and Prevelle® Silk (made by Mentor).

Not all hyaluronic acids are created equal. They differ by source (animal vs. bacterial), by crosslinking, and by modification. In their natural states, hyaluronic acids have poor biomechanical properties as dermal filler. Because hyaluronic acid molecules are highly water soluble, when injected under the skin in their natural states, they clear away in no time. Chemical modification is therefore required to lift the face and to fill wrinkles. Crosslinkers are the most commonly used device to make the product resistant to degradation; the more crosslinked the product, the denser it becomes, making it harder to clear from the body. Most hyaluronic acid fillers boast longevity beyond that of collagen-based dermal fillers; for this reason and also because of problems with allergic reactions, collagen-based fillers are no longer used or preferred.

Restylane and Perlane (made by Galderma Laboratories USA) are non-animal stabilized hyaluronic acids that have been used outside the United States since 1996 and were finally introduced and approved by the FDA in December 2003. Perlane has a higher viscosity because it has larger particles and more crosslinks. In my practice, I use Perlane to improve the volume of the midface and the nasolabial folds after lifting the midface. The perfect patient for this product is someone relatively young (late twenties to forties) who has minimal volume loss or deep nasolabial folds.

Since this product is thick, only a very little product is needed to do a nice correction, making it very cost-effective filler. Perlane is known to last anywhere from nine to twelve months. Restylane is great for augmenting lips and filling fine wrinkles. With dilution to make it less viscous, it also can be safely injected for the treatment of hollow eyes. I do not recommend using the product in this way without diluting it first. As the skin around the eyes is extremely thin, and because the product tends to reflect a blue color (known as the blue Rayleigh effect), people with light or thin skin can appear as if they had dark circles around their eyes.

Restylane typically lasts from three to six months. Its durability in the lips (as with most other lip products) is shorter because the constant movement of the mouth mobilizes the product and speeds up its reabsorption.

Restylane-L® and Perlane-L® are now available. The L indicates that the product contains lidocaine, which is used to increase patient comfort and to decrease the amount of swelling.

Juvéderm Ultra and Juvéderm Ultra Plus (made by Allergan), which were first approved in the United States in 2006, are non-animal stabilized hyaluronic acids that tend to be a lot smoother than their predecessors. A unique method for crosslinking their molecules makes them less granular and longer lasting.

The difference between Juvéderm Ultra and Juvéderm Ultra Plus is the degree of crosslinking. Juvéderm Ultra has a 6-percent degree of crosslinking in its formulation, making it ideal filler for moderate facial wrinkles. In my practice, I tend to use it for filling wrinkles in the forehead, to reduce the appearance of crow's feet. Although Juvéderm Ultra does not result in a blue Rayleigh effect it can look a bit greenish under the eyes. Sometimes this effect is mistakenly referred to as Tyndall effect, but the Tyndall effect involves larger particles. Since most of us have greenish looking veins around our eyes, it does not look unnatural. However, caution is necessary when injecting this product under the eyes of people with allergies or who get puffy eyes in the morning because the product can absorb the fluid and permanently expand. For this reason, I no longer use Juvéderm under the eyes.

Juvéderm Ultra Plus, with its 8-percent degree of crosslinking and robust, 20-percent thicker gel, is ideal for severe folds and for replenishing volume depletion. I use this product mainly to augment lips, and to this day I have found no better product for beautiful, natural-looking smooth lips that last anywhere from six to nine months.

Juvéderm Ultra XC and Juvéderm Ultra Plus XC were recently introduced to the market. The XC stands for "extra comfort." These two formulations contain small amounts of lidocaine that increase patients' comfort and help to reduce swelling. On October 23, 2013, Allergan introduced Juvéderm Voluma® XCTM in the United States, where it became the newest kid on the block in the world of hyaluronic acid-containing fillers. It is the only FDA-approved filler that instantly adds volume and lift to the cheeks with very little product. It creates a more natural and youthful profile, with effects that last for up to two years.

Juvéderm Voluma is an improvement upon the preceding Juvéderm formulations due to the Vycross™ technology used in its manufacture, which produces an efficiently and tightly cross-linked gel that contributes to its lift capacity and its longevity. In my opinion, this product is more appropriate for lifting than for creating volume. This is the reason why the technique we do in my practice with this product is called Rejuva-lift[SM]: It makes the skin appear much more lifted and tighter. Basically, this is the look people usually tell me they want during their intake consultations with me. They usually pull up on the skin around their cheekbones with their fingertips, mildly altering their appearance, and say: "If I could only look like this." The look they desire is pretty much what you get when we do the Rejuva-lift with Juvéderm Voluma.

Prevelle Silk is one of the newest additions of non-animal stabilized hyaluronic acids in my arsenal. It was the first FDA-approved hyaluronic acid that contained lidocaine. I call this product "tryout lips," because it is wonderful for patients who are curious, but not quite sure, about whether or not they want to augment their lips. This product is not as crosslinked as other hyaluronic acids, so it does not last as long. I have many patients, however, who prefer its subtleness and the comfort of its administration.

Belotero Balance® (made by Merz Aesthetics, Inc.), one of the newest approved line fillers in the United States, is a non-animal stabilized hyaluronic acid with a cohesive polydensified matrix that gives this product a unique elasticity. Although there are different formulations of this product in Europe, only the line filler has been approved in the United States as a medical device. "Belotero Soft," as it is called abroad, is ideal for the correction of superficial wrinkles and can be used safely for crow's feet and for perioral and forehead wrinkles.

I love using this product to correct superficial wrinkles. Unlike its predecessors, which must be placed deep enough to hide the product from view, the elasticity of Belotero means that you have more placement options. When used as line filler, Belotero gives better and smoother corrections than all of the hyaluronic acids that came before it.

## RADIESSE (CALCIUM HYDROXYLAPATITE)

Radiesse® (made by Bioform Medical) is injectable filler that was FDA approved in December 2007. It contains calcium hydroxylapatite, a naturally occurring mineral that gives support and strength to bones and teeth. Up to 50 percent of bone is made up of a modified form of this inorganic mineral. Hydroxylapatite can be used as filler for vocal cord insufficiency or to replace amputated bone. It can also be used as a coating to promote bone ingrowth for prosthetic implants, to correct volume depletion, and to improve folds and wrinkles.

This product generated a buzz in Europe in 2004 under the name of Radiance™. The calcium hydroxyapatite in Radiesse is manmade and not taken from cadavers or any other organic source. Since this product is a common mineral that is found in the body, there is no need to test for allergic reactions; however, a person may still be allergic to a component of the formula. For this reason, patients with a history of severe allergic reactions or anaphylaxis should not use this product.

It was first approved in the United States to alleviate the

signs and symptoms of HIV-associated facial lipoatrophy—in other words, the fat loss responsible for the gaunt appearance HIV patients often develop. Even though facial lipoatrophy is not life threatening, it is the most stigmatizing and frustrating complication of HIV. This disease has demonstrated how facial fat is a key ingredient in the fountain of youth. People suffering from this condition can look years older than their chronological ages, even if they are doing quite well in the health department. This can cause severe emotional distress and agony in patients suffering from HIV because it robs them of their self-confidence and quality of life. Radiesse is a blessing in the lives of HIV patients because it provides an immediate and long-lasting correction of this affliction.

During my dermatology residency, I had plenty of opportunities to use this product with HIV patients and fell in love with it. I was able to see, right before my eyes, how it transformed their faces, restoring them to their natural state.

Radiesse was the product that helped me to understand the aging face, as it taught me the importance of volume restoration in turning back the clock. For this reason, I am very fond of Radiesse, and it's one of the most used injectable fillers in my practice. I usually use it to rebuild the cheeks and for other areas of volume depletion. I also use it to improve hollow temples and aging hands, and to reshape noses. It is a versatile product— what you see is what you get!

It is my product of choice for anyone who has facial asymmetry due to volume loss on one side of his or her face. It not only restores the volume loss, but also brings back symmetry and balance, thereby creating a more attractive face.

As filler, Radiesse works very differently from hyaluronic acids, fats, and collagen. It actually works more like the silicones—except that it is not permanent. Introducing calcium hydroxylapatite under the skin will cause a foreign body reaction similar to what we learned with the silicone oils. The body will start laying down new collagen around the molecule to encapsulate the product.

Since the human body knows what to do with calcium, this product degrades quickly, leaving only the patient's newly formed collagen behind. This collagen mimics the volume that was previously given by facial fat, thus lifting and improving the arches and convexities to that of a youthful face. In most cases, the volume correction lasts anywhere from nine to eighteen months, depending on how much product was used, the patient's unique ability to metabolize collagen, and the product itself.

In my practice, we use Radiesse to create beautiful, high cheekbones for women, like those of Kim Kardashian and Jennifer Lopez. This simple technique, which we call HD Sculpt℠, makes anyone appear younger, and it also helps to lift the midface. Many of our patients who love this technique are models— or want to look like one. Well-defined cheekbones can create a dramatic, yet subtle change in a man's face as well. It helps to preserve the contour of the neck and the jawline in a man whose face is starting to descend.

## SCULPTRA AESTHETIC (INJECTABLE POLY-L-LACTIC ACID)

Sculptra Aesthetic (made by Galderma) is a synthetic, biodegradable poly-L-lactic acid-based sugar similar to the material used in absorbable sutures. While similar to silicones, it only hangs around under the skin for about two months. During that period, the body creates a foreign body-like reaction in an attempt to engulf and encapsulate the product. The end result is a volumetric expansion of new collagen and elastic fibers that counteracts the volume loss from bone and fat. Because this product stays under the skin for a couple months before degrading, it creates much more collagen than Radiesse, but less than silicones. Clinical trials have shown that Sculptra corrections are maintained for up to twenty-four months after the last treatment session.

Sculptra was first approved by the FDA in August 2004 for patients with facial lipoatrophy secondary to HIV infection. This product contains a long-lasting bulking agent that has resulted in improved physical appearance, increased self-confidence, and a better quality of life.

For years, dermatologists and plastic surgeons used this phenomenal off-label filler on healthy patients who wanted more durable—though not permanent—filler. In August 2009, Sculptra was finally approved for cosmetics for individuals seeking long-lasting filler for the correction of shallow to deep nasolabial folds, wrinkles, and contour deficiencies.

Before its approval, I was already in love with this product. I call it the smart filler for women because it not only addresses the volume loss in an aging face, it also increases the amount of collagen and elastic fibers in the skin. In addition, it corrects and restores the loss of skeletal structure that accompanies age and menopause.

As mentioned before, Sculptra causes a volumetric expansion of collagen and elastic fibers that counteracts the volume loss from fat. Though both genders are affected by volume loss, only women have to contend with the effects of menopause, which causes their skin to thin and dry out, as well as decreasing the facial bone mass of the mandible. Sculptra addresses many of the perimenopausal and postmenopausal afflictions that rob women of their youthful attributes.

After their treatments with Sculptra, many patients have noticed that their skin feels thicker, more supple, and luminous. This result is secondary to the biostimulation of collagen and elastic fibers that Sculptra induces in the skin. Around menopause, a woman's skin starts to break down more collagen and elastic fibers than it can create, causing the skin to become very thin, dry, and dull. The dullness is an optical effect caused by a lack of sufficient collagen. Collagen has a similar (if not equivalent) molecular size and weight to some of the wavelengths that we find in nature and those that are manmade. When two objects have the same molecular size and weight, they bounce against each other and scatter.

Skin treated with Sculptra creates so much new collagen and elastic fibers that light bounces back off the skin, making it appear luminous. When a person has little collagen and elastic fibers, the light is absorbed into the skin, causing it to appear dull. A luminous skin not only looks healthy and younger, it also makes it difficult for others to perceive the flaws on it. The pores appear smaller, and fine wrinkles and small scars become almost invisible to the naked eye. The opposite is observed in a skin that absorbs light: the pores look larger and every little flaw is magnified.

Part of the aging process is bone remodeling. Unfortunately, due to menopause, women are prone to osteopenia and osteoporosis. Though not as significant an issue for most men, it is a serious matter with serious consequences if ignored for women. These conditions cause a decrease in bone mass in women's hips and legs, as well as in their craniofacial skeletons. For women who are serious about age prevention, it is important to do everything in your power to preserve bone mass. I recommend regular checkups with a primary care provider, doing weight-bearing exercises, and supplementing your diet with calcium, magnesium, and vitamin D3.

Craniofacial bone loss occurs mainly in the upper and lower jaw. Bone loss in the upper jaw is evidenced by an increase in the distance from the corner of the nose to the upper lip. This increase in distance is the result of a loss in volume from the bony elements of the maxilla, leading to a decrease of the available support for the soft tissue in this region. This area tends to look longer, causing the upper lip to roll back into the mouth and decrease in size.

In the lower jawbone, the mandible, we see a more pronounced problem. As it moves inward, it causes the skin and soft tissue above it to collapse into the space formed from the thinning of the bone mass. This is why so many women have such an incredibly hard time maintaining a youthful appearance around their mouths.

Sculptra to the rescue! Sculptra has been an extraordinary solution to correct and prevent this from happening around the mouth. All of my patients have been pleasantly surprised with the corrections and improvements from this product. Sculptra rebuilds the architecture, mimicking with collagen the volume that was once given by the bony structures around the mouth. Although not clinically proven, it is my opinion that it may also help restore the bony elements of the craniofacial skeleton in much the same way that it biostimulates the skin to increase its supply of collagen and elastic fibers. I tell my patients that it's like plastering a wall: It helps maintain bone structure and keeps this problematic area looking youthful.

There is a learning curve when using this product, so I must stress the importance of using a provider who has had plenty of experience using Sculptra. This product should not be injected too superficially into the skin, the red area of the lip, or into areas of a lot of facial movement, such as around the eyes or into the muscles close to the mouth. Although I do use Sculptra on the area above the upper lip, I use a much-diluted form of it to thicken the skin—not to increase the volume. This helps prevent and alleviate the vertical lines above the upper lip and shortens the distance from the corner of the nose to the upper lip. This technique also makes the upper lip appear larger by rolling it back out of the mouth. In addition, it can lift the tip of the nose, which tends to descend and point downward with age, by injecting it at the base of the nose.

Since it is an inert product, an allergy test is not necessary when using Sculptra. That being said, any patient with a known allergy to any of the product's ingredients or with a history of severe allergic reactions should not use this product. In addition, people with a history of keloid formation or hypertrophic scars, or who have an autoimmune disease, are not candidates for this product. Patients with permanent cheek or chin implants should notify their providers in order to prevent a possible infection or simply to avoid these areas. Lastly, Sculptra should never be injected into areas where silicones or other permanent fillers have been injected in the past.

The most common side effects encountered with the use of Sculptra in my practice are mild swelling and bruising. We recommend that all our patients take bromelain (pineapple enzyme) five days prior to the procedure and homeopathic *Arnica montana* on the day of the procedure to prevent swelling and bruising.

Nodules sometimes form under the skin with delayed onset; however, these tend to resolve by themselves. For this reason, I hydrate the Sculptra for more than twenty-four hours in advance to turn it into a fine liquid. This prevents an exuberant foreign body reaction to larger particles of the product, which can result in nodule formation.

In contrast to other fillers, the results of Sculptra are not typically apparent immediately after a procedure. The improvements that some patients notice after the procedure are mainly from water and inflammation. Two days later, it often looks as if no treatment has even been done. Patients are advised to massage the treated area five times a day, for five minutes, for five days. I usually tell them to remember the fictitious phone number in the movies that always starts with "555."

The final results of the procedure will be appreciated about eight weeks later. It requires multiple treatments, and while every patient is different, the average in my clinic is two sessions using two vials per session.

I recommend that older and vegetarian patients drink a protein shake as a snack once a day to ensure that they have enough building blocks in their bodies to make more collagen. I came to this conclusion after observing what happens to me when I work out and don't drink protein shakes—I simply can't bulk up. You need protein to make protein! I also noticed that my older and vegetarian patients do not fill up as well as younger ones with more nutritionally balanced diets. Since I have been recommending protein shakes, however, I have noticed that they respond just as well or better.

I began by using Sculptra as a skin thickener, but when patients started to return to my practice after I had used it to rebuild volume I saw miraculous changes in their faces. I went from using a couple of vials of Sculptra a month to becoming the #1 user in the nation, a distinction that I maintain to this day.

The name of the technique I developed with Sculptra Aesthetic is Precise-Sculpt[SM], because the filler is injected with precision into the areas of the facial bones that change with the passing of time. Over time, the Sculptra stimulates collagen formations that imitate natural bone, fat, and collagen in the skin. My technique has been so successful that I spend my free time teaching it to my residents and other colleagues in the aesthetics and cosmetic dermatology field.

## AUTOLOGOUS PLASMA INJECTIONS

I went to Bogota, Colombia, in September 2009 to train a few doctors in a new laser technology called Affirm Multiplex and to attend a media event with Alejandro Rada Cassab, M.D., one of the most renowned and respected physicians in the world of aesthetics. While visiting his state of the art facility, the Rada Cassab Medicina Estetica, I was astonished to learn a new and clever technique for replenishing volume using a patient's own blood. I felt like I was in the movie set for the 1992 film *Death Becomes Her* with Meryl Streep and Goldie Hawn. I watched with fascination as a patient watched as her blood was drawn from her arm. Upon seeing my confused expression, Dr Rada Cassab explained that he was going to extract platelet-rich plasma from the patient's blood in order to use it as filler. Since I had never heard of such a procedure, I asked him to enlighten me with all the details.

The entire procedure takes thirty to forty-five minutes and causes little discomfort. Blood is drawn from the patient at the time of the procedure and is prepared in the clinic by centrifuge. The plasma, which is rich in epidermal growth factors and platelets, is then injected in the same manner that hyaluronic acid is customarily used. The beauty of this procedure is that the patient's own blood is used, so the risk of an allergic reaction is nonexistent.

Additionally, no serious side effects or adverse reactions have been observed using this procedure. This is a smart type of filler because it's autologous (drawn from the individual whom it is going to be used to treat) and full of epidermal growth factors, proteins that help the skin become more luminous and supple. This nutrient-rich filler not only improves mild volume depletion and helps with wrinkles; it also nurtures and improves the skin. The results last about six months, but the texture and quality of the skin last even longer.

This procedure is so effective that even two or more years after its introduction in the United States the cosmetics industry is still buzzing about this "vampire filler."

The Selphyl® System enables for a quick and safe preparation of autologous, platelet-rich plasma and platelet-rich fibrin matrix. It's an in-office procedure in which the patient's blood is drawn and then goes through a centrifugal process to separate the platelet-rich plasma from the red blood cells. The resulting product is then injected into the treatment area similar to hyaluronic acid filler. It has been approved to treat frown lines, nasolabial folds, acne scars, and sunken eyes. The beauty of this product is that you can never over correct with it. In addition, it stimulates collagen production to create a volumetric expansion in the skin matrix that helps to fill in wrinkles and improve the loss of volume over time.

The technology used to create vampire filler is not new at all. I know for a fact that orthopedic surgeons in the United States have been using the same procedure to treat chronic tendonitis, muscle fibrosis, and ligament injuries as an alternative to cortisone injections, with excellent results. The growth factors in the platelet-rich injections stimulate a healing response in damaged tissue. In my practice, we have introduced a new technique, Stem-Scalp Essence[SM], which utilizes platelet-rich plasma (PRP) to regrow hair. We are seeing excellent results when the patients' own PRP is injected into their scalps.

This is the beginning of a new era of regenerative medicine in which scientists, engineers, biologists, chemists, and physicians are joining forces to create a natural microenvironment that encourages the healing and regeneration of damaged tissue. Body, heal thyself!

## AUTOLOGOUS MATURE STEM CELLS PLUS FAT INJECTIONS

This new technique, a hybrid of the traditional fat transfer method and autologous plasma injections, helps patients maintain the arches and convexities of a youthful face. As I mentioned earlier, fat transfer has been around for a long time as an efficient way to restore volume in the face. However, the results can be unpredictable. Up to 50 percent of the harvested fat cells die after they have been injected into the recipient site. Due to this well-known disadvantage, most physicians tend to overfill their patients, leaving them looking overstuffed until the transferred fats settle down a few months later.

Recently, a new technique to restore facial volume with autologous fat plus mature stem cells has proven to be a very effective procedure. Since stem cells have the innate capability to develop into any kind of tissue or organ, when they are added during a fat transfer, the stem cells nurture and maintain the newly transferred fat cells, thereby enabling more of them to live. Instead of losing almost half of the fat cells after being transferred, only 5–10 percent of the grafted fats perish.

The procedure is done under local anesthesia, and the fat is harvested via liposuction from the lower abdomen. A total volume of about a quarter of a liter of fat is extracted, half of it being used to harvest the stem cells. A device called the Celution® System processes the fat tissue and liberates the stem and regenerative cells. The cells are then collected using a syringe and recombined with the other half of the extracted fat. This stem cell-rich fat is then used in areas that show volume depletion. This new stem cell-rich and regenerative cell-rich matrix under the skin both enhances volume and makes the skin more luminous, toned, and elastic.

This new technique reveals and validates what I have been professing to my patients for years: Fat is a key ingredient in the fountain of youth.

CHAPTER 9

# Rays of Light

Laser light technology has been one of the most innovative and exciting advancements in medicine and aesthetic surgery in recent years. Growing up, I remember watching sci-fi movies and thinking that lasers were powerful and mystical, but something far off in the future. In movies, they were mostly used as weapons, such as the light saber in *Star Wars* and the phaser from *Star Trek.*

In actuality, laser technology can be found pretty much everywhere today. Lasers are in supermarkets, dance clubs, CD players, and even in museums, where they are used to clean precious statues and artifacts. We can now add medical and aesthetic applications to the list.

It is amazing to see so many things that were considered sci-fi in my younger years that are now a reality. It is as if yesterday's science fiction has become today's science fact! I am just waiting to say, "Beam me up, Scotty," and get transported to remote areas of the universe in the blink of an eye. Until then, I intend to take full advantage of the age-prevention and age-reversal properties of aesthetic lasers.

The principles of laser technology were first introduced in *The Quantum Theory of Radiation* by Albert Einstein in 1917. Drawing upon Einstein's theory, other scientists began to develop lasers for a variety of purposes. It wasn't until the 1960s, however, that scientists were able to successfully emit a continuous beam of light.

There is a lot of controversy around the question of who invented the first laser. Many believe that Gordon Gould, then a doctoral student at Colombia University (who never received his degree), invented the first optical laser. Although he began building it in 1958, he failed to file a patent for his invention until 1959. Due to this careless mistake, many other scientists exploited his technology and were able to generate different types of optical lasers before him. In fact, it was not until 1977 that Gould received his first patent for a laser. Despite all of the controversy, one fact remains clear: Gordon Gould was the first person ever to use the word laser.

LASER is shorthand for *light amplification by the stimulated emission of radiation*. In this case, *radiation* refers to a radiant body of light—not to the dangerous aftermath of a nuclear power plant meltdown.

Aesthetic lasers are light that is turned into heat. Most structures in the human body get destroyed at temperatures above 40 degrees Celsius. Laser radiation is a nonionizing type of radiation that is distinct from X-rays, UV rays, and gamma rays, all of which can alter human DNA to cause cancer and birth defects. Across the board, no matter what use they are being applied to, lasers have pretty much the same components: a lasing medium that contains electrons in a resting state, a pumping (external) source, and two mirrors. The lasing medium can be a gas, a semi-precious stone (for example, a ruby), or a dye.

When the electrons in the lasing medium absorb light, the energy from an external source (for example, a flash lamp) gets excited and moves up to a higher energy state. Then, the tendency for electrons is always to revert back to their normal resting positions. In the process, they release energy in the form of light. This process occurs multiple times at an incredible speed until a bright, colorful beam of light is released from the laser apparatus.

Do you remember learning in Physics 101 that energy in a closed system can neither be created nor destroyed, but is always being transformed into something else? That's the first law of thermodynamics, the law of conservation. In the case of aesthetic lasers, the energy from the light is transformed mainly into heat, as well as into shock waves and acoustic waves. The best analogy to illustrate a laser is a glow-in-the-dark sticker. In order for the sticker to glow in the dark, it needs to be brought to a source of light.

The sticker itself has a chemical medium that contains electrons in its molecules. The electrons in the medium absorb the energy in the form of light and then move up to an excited state. As they come down to their resting states, energy in the form of a bright light is emitted. The longer you hold the sticker to the source of light, the brighter the sticker becomes after turning off the lights and the longer the light will glow. Who knew that one day this little observation was going to change the world of aesthetics?

Thank you, thank you, thank you, Professor Einstein! Your work continues to bless our lives.

The very first laser to have any clinical significance was the ruby laser introduced by physicist Theodore Maiman, Ph.D., in 1960. Other lasers quickly followed, such as the neodymium-doped yttrium aluminum garnet (Nd:YAG) laser in 1961, the argon laser in 1962, and the carbon dioxide laser in 1964.

Lasers are usually named after the constituents of the laser medium and the type of wavelengths they generate. A laser using a ruby stone as a constituent of the medium, for example, generates a light with a wavelength of 694 nanometers (nm). As you may recall, a nanometer is one-billionth of a meter. Therefore, this laser is known as the 694 nm ruby laser. The laser's wavelength is measured by using a wavelength meter. It ensures that a particular lasing medium is truly putting out the exact wavelength that is purported.

Laser light has specific characteristics that differentiate it from conventional light sources. First off, it is coherent and collimated, meaning that laser light beams travel parallel to each other like soldiers in a marching band. They also can travel long distances while maintaining the same level of energy as when they were first emitted from the machine. For this reason, appropriate eye protection is necessary to avoid getting seriously injured by a laser.

Laser light is also monochromatic—a light of a single color. This means that each laser light has a predilection and an affinity for a specific type of tissue. For example, a 755-nm alexandrite laser has a predilection to destroy anything that is black or brown. Aesthetically we can use this to treat any tissue that contains eumelanin (aka "true" melanin), such as hair and age spots. Pheomelanin, a reddish yellow pigment also found in human hair and skin, is not affected by this wavelength.

The 1064-nm Nd:YAG laser has a predilection for hemoglobin in the red blood cells, so it is useful for destroying spider veins. By contrast, the 1440-nm Nd:YAG laser has an affinity for water in the dermis, so it's fantastic for destroying unwanted collagen and elastic fibers found in scars, stretch marks, and wrinkles. It helps to produce new collagen and elastic fibers that resemble normal skin.

Because of the unique properties of laser light, one can use a particular wavelength to destroy an unwanted lesion on the skin without harming other structures. This process is called selective photothermolysis. If it were not for these laser light characteristics, everyone would be at home removing hair or spider veins with a flashlight.

I am in love with laser light technology and everything that deals with tissue–light interaction. It is fascinating to see how we can use different wavelengths of light either to destroy or to generate various tissues on our skin. We have laser lights that destroy brown spots, red lesions, and unwanted hair and fat. We also have lasers that increase collagen and elastic fibers in our skin. Every year scientists isolate or combine different types of wavelengths to tackle most of the changes that happen to our bodies with age. In the future, I predict that conventional plastic surgery will only exist in the archives of medical literature.

I have been fascinated with laser technology since it was introduced to me when I was an intern in family medicine. I had a burning desire to understand and master this technology so that I could offer it to my future patients. This was the beginning of my pursuit of becoming a cosmetic dermatologist.

There are many different types of laser wavelengths, as well as companies that create them, so it can be confusing for doctors and patients alike. Since the very beginning of the laser revolution, I made it a point to only associate myself with the companies that had the best scientists on board so that I would be able to offer only the highest quality, most reliable technology to my patients. In this type of business, your success is tied to the quality of outcomes that you produce. Most of my laser technology comes from Cynosure, Inc., a company based in Boston. The scientists at Cynosure continuously create safe, effective, and reliable laser technology.

*Note:* Although in this section I am using the names of the tools utilized in my practice, your doctor may get similar results as the ones I describe while using a different brand of laser technology, as long as the devices produce the same wavelengths of light as the ones described below.

In the next section, I will discuss the lasers that I use in my practice, including their wavelengths, lasing mediums, and applications. It is my personal experience—and I believe that my patients would concur—that the laser technology I am about to discuss has consistently delivered on what it has promised.

Before beginning our discussion on laser technology, it is important to mention that not all laser wavelengths are appropriate for all skin tones and types. In order to avoid adverse reactions, it is important to match the right wavelength with the right skin tone. This can be achieved by classifying patients by their skin types.

Fitzpatrick Skin Types is the classification system most commonly used by dermatologists to predict which of their patients will be prone to photoaging and skin cancer. It has also been helpful in selecting the appropriate wavelength for the laser that will treat a particular skin tone.

---

## A QUICK REFERENCE GUIDE TO FITZPATRICK SKIN TYPES

- **Type I:** Always burns, never tans, has light-colored hair and eyes (Caucasian, possibly Scandinavian in heritage).
- **Type II:** Usually burns, tans with difficulty, and has light skin and blue or light-colored eyes (Caucasian, possibly Irish or German in heritage).
- **Type III:** Sometimes burns, but usually tans, has eyes darker in color, and slight coloring of the skin (possibly Northern Mediterranean or Asian in heritage).
- **Type IV:** Rarely burns, tans easily, has dark eye coloring and skin color (possibly Spanish or Native American heritage).
- **Type V:** Very rarely burns, has dark hair and eye color (possibly of Southern Indian or Spanish-African heritage).
- **Type VI:** Has very dark skin, dark coarse hair, and dark eyes (of African heritage).

---

Skin types I, II, and III are usually more prone to sun damage and premature aging. Skin types IV, V, and VI are darker complexions that tend to withstand more sun exposure. However, darker complexions require more precaution in selecting the appropriate laser wavelength that will respect their skin tones.

## HAIR LASERS

We have a love-hate relationship with hair in our society. We want it on our scalps, eyelashes, and brows, but despise it almost anywhere else on our bodies. It is amazing to see how our obsession with this structure, composed primarily of dead protein, has become a multibillion-dollar industry. We do so many different things with our hair: from changing its color, texture, and shape to making personal statements about our individuality. Hair can even express sexual energy, which is why some religions prohibit women from showing their manes in public.

A multitude of laser and light devices are used for the depilation of hair. So many, in fact, that it can get confusing trying to choose the right laser to destroy the hair follicles without harming the skin. This confusion, besides being felt by consumers, is also felt by the practitioners purchasing and operating the devices.

During my seminars, I like to give information about laser light technology based on the specifications of individual wavelengths. In order to destroy hair, a wavelength that has an affinity for true melanin (brown/black pigment) must be utilized. Since so many devices claim that they will get the job done, I like to stress which of the available wavelengths is the most efficient for a particular Fitzpatrick skin type. For example, if you have skin type I, II, or III, there is nothing better and safer than a 755-nm wavelength alexandrite laser, or "Alex." Skin types I–III tend to have finer and lighter hairs, containing less melanin. The 755-nm Alex is the gold standard for hair removal for people with lighter skin and fine hair at the present time.

If your skin type is in the range of IV–VI, the safest wavelength to destroy hair—while still respecting your skin—is the 1064-nm wavelength, the Nd:YAG. The 1064-nm wavelength does not have as much affinity for melanin as the 755-nm laser, meaning it will not go for the melanin that is found in the skin.

People that naturally look tan or dark have structures under their skin called melanosomes that tend to be larger in darker skin types than in lighter ones. These are like little bubbles containing melanin. If you use a wavelength that has a lot of affinity for melanin, it will go for both the melanin in the hair and in the skin. The 1064-nm wavelength will only go for the hair if the hair is coarse and thick, making it ideal for use on individuals of African and Latino descent.

Only hair that is actively growing (in the anagen phase) can be destroyed by laser light. It is an absolute miracle that 85 percent of all hairs on the human body are actively growing from head to toe. If it wasn't for this miracle, depilation via laser hair removal could not be possible. The hair shaft that is actively growing is attached to the hair follicle and attracts the light because it contains melanin in its shaft. The laser light travels down the hair shaft to the area where the cells that make up the hair structure reside. The laser turns up the heat of the follicle to 40 degrees Celsius and basically cooks it until it perishes.

Since not all of the hairs are actively growing in one area, multiple treatments are required. The hair cells that are in other phases of their lifecycle (the catagen, or cessation phases; and the telogen, or resting, phase) do not have their hair shafts attached to the follicle, and hence, will survive the laser treatment. The good news is that hair transitions from one phase to another; eventually, most hairs will be eliminated. Although this treatment leads to a permanent hair reduction, patients need to understand that there may be a regrowth of some hair due to a genetic predisposition to having a lot of body hair. Patient satisfaction, however, is generally high with laser depilation treatment.

There is not a good wavelength at this moment to treat platinum blond, gray, white, or red hair with lasers. These patients would need to utilize other processes for depilation, such as electrolysis, waxing, or plucking. In my practice, I use the Apogee® Elite and Apogee Elite MPX lasers (made by Cynosure, Inc.) for hair removal because they use the two gold standard wavelengths, 755 nm and 1064 nm, to destroy hair efficiently without harming the skin. The specifications of the Apogee Elite lasers allow me to treat almost anyone who walks into my clinic and gain superior results in a relatively short amount of time.

## VASCULAR LESIONS

Vascular lesions can arise shortly after birth like a port wine stain, or they can be acquired like the facial and leg veins that come with age or during pregnancy. Superficial vascular lesions have a bright red appearance; deep vascular lesions tend to be more bluish. Lesions of color on the skin are considered competing chromophores, meaning that they compete to absorb light and can make the skin look dull or sallow, as well as magnify any skin flaws.

The therapy for vascular lesions uses the principle of selective photothermolysis, in which a laser light has an affinity for the hemoglobin content inside blood vessels—yet for nothing else around it. The blood vessels get heated up above 65 degrees Celsius and are basically cooked in the process. The body then starts absorbing the necrotic (dying) tissue and the blood vessels begin to vanish. Since hemoglobin is an essential element in red blood cells, vascular lasers treat most red lesions on the skin, such as hemangiomas, port wine stains, red stretch marks, rosacea, psoriasis, and varicose veins.

There are many different wavelengths that have an affinity for vascular lesions; however some are superior and safer than others. The gold standard wavelength for vascular lesions is that emitted by the pulsed dye laser (PDL), which has a wavelength ranging from 585-595 nm. As the name suggests, PDLs use a liquid dye, usually rhodamine 64, which produces a yellow light. This yellow light laser targets the red to brown color spectrum and is usually used to treat very bright red and superficial vascular lesions. The problem with this wavelength is that in order to get great results, patients may acquire bruises in the treatment areas. However, newer versions of this laser exist that have considerably reduced the incidence of bruising.

Since the 1064-nm wavelength is a light that tends to penetrate deeply, it is ideal for varicose lesions on the legs. The 1064-nm Nd:YAG is also great to remove the little blood vessels that tend to form around the nose, chin, and cheeks. The beauty of this wavelength is that there is no risk of bruising to the patient. No downtime is therefore necessary for recovery. Only someone who is experienced should treat varicose veins, and it usually requires two or three sessions to achieve the desired results.

In my practice, I use the 1064-nm wavelength Apogee Elite MPX laser for small varicose veins in the legs and for little hemangiomas and facial telangiectasias (spider veins). In addition to the Apogee Elite MPX, I use the Cynergy laser, which offers both 595-nm (PDL) and 1064-nm (Nd:YAG) wavelengths in a multiplex technology. Multiplex (MPX) technology is unique in that it provides what I like to call the "double whammy effect." It uses both gold standard wavelengths for vascular lesions, simultaneously. The 595-nm PDL shoots first and is followed within milliseconds by the Nd:YAG 1064-nm wavelength. Because two wavelengths with different affinities for blood vessels are being used, less energy from either wavelength is needed to accomplish the job. This translates into a safer, more comfortable, and more effective treatment.

There is one other wavelength used for vascular lesions worth mentioning: the 532-nm wavelength (KTP). This wavelength is obtained by adding potassium titanyl phosphate crystal to the 1064-nm Nd:YAG crystal. This creates a green light with a greater affinity for hemoglobin. This wavelength is great for facial telangiectasias because it heats up the blood vessels without causing any bruising.

## PHOTOAGING AND WRINKLES

Since the introduction of laser light in the aesthetics world, scientists and doctors keep finding new laser light applications to aid in the rejuvenation and contouring of the face with virtually no downtime for recovery. Most of the laser light procedures that are used these days are geared to rebuild the scaffold of the skin, the dermis, using new collagen and elastic fibers. This both tightens redundant, saggy skin and eliminates any blemishes on the surface of the skin.

In my practice, we offer different types of photofacials in order to meet the needs of our clientele. Nonablative laser treatments often leave the skin a little flush for a few hours, while other laser treatments make someone look like an Oompa Loompa for a few days. The term *nonablative* refers to lasers that do not burn the top layer of the skin. These lasers generate heat deep below the skin to stimulate new collagen formation. There are also more aggressive ablative laser photofacials that burn the top layer of the skin, making someone's skin look like hamburger meat. Understandably, most people avoid this type of laser treatment because it comes with a lengthy downtime period. However, research has shown that the results of the ablative lasers are much more impressive than any other laser.

The laser light procedures that we offer in my practice to rejuvenate the skin use wavelengths that destroy old, sun-damaged collagen and elastic fibers. They also stimulate new collagen and elastic fibers, tighten the skin and eliminate brown or red discoloration on the skin. We are also using a laser light that has the capability to shrink sagging tissue, giving a more toned texture to a skin that has lost its elasticity from aging, smoking, or sun damage.

Since we offer a plethora of photofacials in our practice, I will mention the different lasers used for skin rejuvenation, starting with the mildest and moving to the strongest. Keep in mind that such lasers work by generating heat under the skin. The skin senses the heat and responds to the injury by laying down new collagen and elastic fibers to repair itself. Stronger lasers have a longer downtime, but they also provide more spectacular results.

My formula to match the right patient with the right wavelength is simple. First of all, I look at the skin tone of the patient to determine the most compatible wavelength. Second, I look at the degree of sun damage and the levels of intrinsic and extrinsic aging. If the patient is young and starting to show signs of premature wrinkling or mild sun damage, I choose a nonablative laser. If the patient is older or has severe sun damage, I like to bring out the "big gun": an ablative laser. Last, I always find out what the patient's expectations are, including how much time he or she is willing to commit to the healing process.

## APOGEE ELITE PHOTOFACIAL

The Apogee Elite (Cynosure, Inc.) photofacial is for the younger patient population who want their skin to look a bit brighter—especially the women who want to start increasing their bank account of collagen and elastic fibers. It is also useful for patients with active acne or blemishes. The wavelength is the 1064-nm Nd:YAG. This photofacial will even out skin tone, brighten the skin, and help prevent wrinkles. The same wavelength can be used at a higher setting for tissue tightening. Since it is a mild, nonablative photofacial, it is not a good choice for very mature or sun-damaged skin. The 1064 nm is a great wavelength to treat skin of color and to help even out blemishes and other types of discoloration.

## CYNERGY MULTIPLEX PHOTOFACIAL

Cynergy Multiplex (Cynosure, Inc.) is another nonablative pho-tofacial. I generally use it with patients who have red undertones on their skin, rosacea, seborrhea, psoriasis, or mottled skin. It is wonderful because it generates collagen and elastic fibers, and it also evens out skin tone. This laser has the advantage of having two wavelengths shooting at once, thus targeting many flaws on the skin with one treatment. It is a little more aggres-sive than the Apogee Elite photofacial. The 595-nm wavelength, in combination with the 1064-nm wavelength, ensures that any vascular lesions on the skin get eliminated. The 1064-nm wave-length has tissue-tightening capabilities, and the 595-nm wave-length has an affinity for red and brown lesions. The heat gener-ated by both wavelengths stimulates fibroblast cells to lay down new collagen and elastic fibers.

## INTENSE PULSED LIGHT PHOTOFACIAL

Intense pulsed light (IPL) devices usually utilize a potent xenon flash lamp that generates a white light with a multitude of wave-lengths (560 nm–1200 nm) from the visible light spectrum. Fil-ters are used in order to make an IPL device behave like a laser, even though it does not naturally do so. An IPL device emits multiple wavelengths of different colors, making it polychromat-ic, divergent, and noncoherent.

This means that an IPL is everything that a laser is not. I love laser and light technology, but I find IPLs useful in removing sun-spots, very superficial red spots, and fine wrinkles and in treat-ing acne. Since there are multiple wavelengths generated from an IPL, multiple superficial targets in the skin can be treated with one device. In my practice, we use Palomar IPL technolo-gy (Cynosure, Inc.) to activate Levulan® (aminolevulinic acid), a chemical used for the treatment of pre-skin cancers with photo-dynamic therapy, and to treat diffuse mottled skin.

## PHOTODYNAMIC THERAPY

It amazes me that we can actually use light to reverse photodam-age and to prevent and treat pre-skin cancers. I can say without reservation that UV rays from sunlight cause most of the wrin-kles, discoloration, and skin cancers that we see in the general population. Fortunately, technology has advanced to the point that we are able to harvest different types of lights to counter-act the harmful effects of past chronic sunlight exposure.

Nowadays, we are using light to treat the adverse effects of light, just as firefighters use fire to control wildfires. In my prac-tice, we use two different wavelengths in combination with a solution of aminolevulinic acid to treat and prevent precursors of skin cancer. Levulan, the brand name for aminolevulinic acid, is a light sensitizing drug that, when activated, seeks and destroys rapidly dividing cells in precancerous lesions. It also improves moderate to severe acne. There is a new photosensitizer with the brand name, Allumera®, which can be activated by red and blue light for facial rejuvenation, shrinking pores, acne, and rosacea.

We use the Omnilux Blue™ and the Omnilux Revive™ to treat mild to moderate acne and to activate the aminolevulinic acid. The Omnilux™ light technology was developed after twelve years of intense medical research on light–tissue interactions. This technology, based on narrowband light-emitting diodes (LEDs), is used for a variety of dermatological conditions, such as acne, vitiligo, hair loss, non-melanoma skin cancers, pho-todamage, and wound healing.

The Omnilux Blue generates a narrowband, blue wavelength of 415 nm that activates the aminolevulinic acid for photody-namic treatment of pre-skin cancers. In addition, this wave-length targets acne-causing bacteria, making the bacteria's own secretions toxic for them without harming the skin or body.

The Omnilux Revive generates a narrowband red wavelength of 633 nm that also activates aminolevulinic acid. This wavelength penetrates deep under the skin, resulting in a more exuberant reaction when treating superficial, non-melanoma skin cancers. I call this wavelength my "miracle light" because it speeds up the natural healing process of the body. For patients who bruise easily, this light will improve the bruising and inflammation within one day. I also use it to improve and heal leg ulcers, rosacea, and inflammatory acne.

Clinical studies have clearly demonstrated that the 633-nm red light enhances DNA synthesis and augments cellular tissue regeneration pathways, including collagen deposition. There are now devices with this red light that stimulate hair growth and serve as an over-the-counter handheld comb. This means people can now treat their own hair loss at home. The expense of these devices varies. In addition, this red LED light is effective in increasing the amount of collagen and elastic fibers under the skin via photomodulation.

Another treatment application for this red light is for vitiligo. This depigmentation condition causes reduced levels of the enzyme catalase, which leads to an increased concentration of hydrogen peroxide in the skin. The hydrogen peroxide interferes with the activity of another enzyme, tyrosinase, which is important for the production of melanin pigment. When using the red light together with a salve of pseudocatalase, the levels of hydrogen peroxide begin to decrease and tyrosinase begins its work of making normal skin pigment.

*Note:* the short wavelength of the red and blue light devices can cause the condition of any patient with melasma to worsen.

## AFFIRM MULTIPLEX PHOTOFACIAL

The Affirm MultiPlex (made by Cynosure, Inc.) is a 1440-nm and 1320-nm wavelength dual-laser light technology that destroys damaged collagen and elastic fibers and slowly replaces them with new collagen and elastic fibers. It simultaneously tightens the skin by shrinking subcutaneous tissue (3–5 millimeters per treatment) with virtually no downtime. This equates to patients being able to go back to work the next day. We find unwanted collagen and elastic fibers, known as solar elastosis, in photodamaged skin, as well as in scars, stretch marks, and keloids (irregularly shaped scars). This wavelength is therefore not only useful in improving and eliminating wrinkles, but also helps blend unsightly scars.

When the skin gets injured, the body starts the healing process immediately to prevent infection. It begins to repair the injured site by laying down a type of collagen that is made in a hurry. Unfortunately, it doesn't look or feel like the rest of the skin. This is why scars often have a different texture and are visible. The 1440-nm wavelength destroys the abnormal collagen, and within four to six weeks starts to replace it with newer collagen that looks like the rest of the skin. In a recent study that one of my residents and I conducted at our practice, we were able to significantly improve many keloids—and some even vanished completely.

Another useful application for the 1440-nm wavelength is for the treatment of resistant melasma. There are very few wavelengths that aid in the treatment of this hormone-regulated disease. Most of the existing wavelengths cause the condition to worsen. My personal and professional opinion is that the 1440 nm and 1540 nm are the only wavelengths that improve this condition without the risk of a rebound.

The other wavelength that has tissue-tightening capabilities in this dual laser is the 1320-nm wavelength. The Affirm MultiPlex is the only technology of its kind to combine the 1440-nm wavelength with the 1320-nm wavelength. The 1440 nm helps decrease the amount of wrinkles on the skin, while the 1320 nm tightens it. As a nonablative technology, it does not harm the top layer of the skin and therefore requires little downtime.

## SMARTSKIN $CO_2$ PHOTOFACIAL

The SmartSkin $CO_2$ laser (Cynosure, Inc.) is a microablative laser light that works like the Affirm MultiPlex, but more aggressively, with a downtime of at least three to five days. It can give someone with extremely wrinkled skin or with severe acne scarring a new, suppler, and more even-textured skin. The wavelength of the $CO_2$ laser is 10,600 nm. It is a single laser that is able to resurface sun-damaged skin and rejuvenate collagen all in one treatment. It can treat scars, sun freckles, stretch marks, poor skin texture, and a variety of other challenging skin conditions.

The original $CO_2$ laser, which has been around since the early 1980s, has a lengthy recovery period. The risk for complication is high, and it is only used on people with very light complexions. Although the patient might appear wrinkle-free after treatment, the skin may look extremely white, poreless, and glossy. This unnatural look, combined with the high risk of complications and the prolonged downtime after treatment, have made many people shy away from this technology.

The SmartSkin $CO_2$ microablative technology recently emerged and has revolutionized the way we treat an aging skin. It has the same $CO_2$ wavelength, but it is delivered by a proprietary scanning system that ablates the skin with microspacing in between normal skin. This treatment gives someone a visibly younger skin in as little as one session with very little downtime. The analogy that I use to compare the old fashioned $CO_2$ and the new microablative delivery system is that the old $CO_2$ laser was like using a blowtorch. The entire surface of the skin was completely burned. With the microablative $CO_2$ technology, however, there are spaces of unharmed normal skin between the areas of the injured skin.

Around the hair follicle, we encounter specialized skin cells that move to areas of skin injury and initiate the healing process. If you use a blowtorch and burn absolutely everything on the skin, including the specialized cells, then the healing process is going to take a very long time. However, by using the microablative technology, plenty of the specialized skin cells are left unharmed to start the healing process.

The old-fashioned $CO_2$ laser took two or more months to heal, while the newer microablative technology takes five to seven days, even if the device is set on the most aggressive settings. With the microablative technology, there is not as much bleeding or oozing, and the skin tone and texture are greatly improved. There isn't the risk of acquiring glossy white, unnatural looking skin, and I am able to use it on patients with light brown skin tones, as well. These days, anyone can have truly beautiful skin at any age.

## SMARTLIPO TRIPLEX

As we age, we lose midface volume and the apples of our faces become more like flat pancakes. We also get fat accumulation around and under our jaw, causing a downward pull of the tissue above and resulting in the gaunt, tired appearance in the face. The Smartlipo Triplex™ (made by Cynosure, Inc.) can be a great alternative to a lower facelift. It achieves unbelievable results by using three combined laser lights that permanently melt fat and tighten skin at the same time.

The results are a nice jawline contour and tighter skin. In addition, by releasing the downward pull of the tissue by removing the excess fat the rest of the face gains elasticity, so the face looks more rested. There is little downtime with this technology, and people can sometimes return to their routine daily activities as early as in a few days.

The Smartlipo Triplex is going to revolutionize the way liposuction is done. Patients these days not only want flat tummies, but a more toned and athletic appearance. Washboard stomachs and a better female waistline are now conceivable with this high definition, laser-assisted lipolysis.

The Smartlipo Triplex uses three different wavelengths to achieve these incredible results. The 1440-nm wavelength that we discussed in the Affirm Multiplex is also used in this device. This miraculous wavelength has forty times greater absorption of fatty tissue than any of the other wavelengths. Since less energy and heat are required to obtain the desired results, there are less thermal injuries. Physicians are able to work safely and effectively in the most superficial layers of fat. The 1440-nm wavelength not only gets rid of unwanted fat by causing thermal injury to the fat cells, but also, mechanically, by creating microbubbles that collapse and cause more disruption of the fat cells.

The Smartlipo Triplex also uses the 1320-nm wavelength, a very hot wavelength that can be used in combination with the 1064-nm wavelength for a more efficient laser-assisted lipolysis and skin tightening. The 1064-nm wavelength coagulates the blood vessels during the procedure, preventing blood loss and discomfort, while the 1320-nm wavelength is extremely efficient in melting undesirable fat.

This technology is also great for physically fit individuals who cannot get the six-pack abs that they want no matter how hard they try. Most people struggle with an area or two of stubborn fat, such as saddlebags, muffin tops, bra fat, or the infamous "love handles." The Smartlipo Triplex obtains high-definition results with only a minor risk of complications.

# CHAPTER 10

# Lotions and Potions

I often get overwhelmed looking at the myriad containers of lotions and potions in department stores that promise the newest and most advanced ingredients in age reversal. There seems always to be a new antioxidant claiming to have that *je ne sais quoi* ingredient du jour from a mysterious plant growing only in a remote area of the world that can prevent the skin from aging. I get overwhelmed, but I also want to try everything, because . . . you never know!

We've made so many great advances in the skin care industry in recent years, from producing better and smarter moisturizers to serums and sunblocks that have antiaging properties. We also understand more about the physiology of the skin and the effects that certain substances have upon it. Using products containing retinoic acid, for example, can increase the amount of collagen in the dermis by activating the retinoic acid receptor (RAR) alpha gene. The more collagen and elastic fibers that are under the surface of the skin, the less likely it is that the skin will wrinkle prematurely.

We've come a long way from using Nivea® or Pond's® creams as our exclusive moisturizers. My grandmother couldn't live without her C and S creams from Pond's, which didn't contain antioxidants or any of the cosmeceutical ingredients that were developed since these products first came to market. I remember taking her creams and mixing them with other ingredients, such as cocoa butter, egg whites, chocolate, and avocados, and telling her that these were good for her skin. She believed me and always tried my concoctions. She'd even tell her friends about the awesome results that she was getting. After all these years, it is only now dawning on me that she may have been trying to make me feel good about my inventions—and it worked, I never stopped being fascinated with skin care.

It might have been a placebo effect, or maybe I really was on to something at the tender age of six. Either way, from an early age I've wanted to create something that would make people look and feel more beautiful.

The cosmetic industry is oversaturated with products that advertise sensational results, but lack the scientific evidence and control studies to back them up. The term *cosmeceutical* is a hybrid word used to represent the union of cosmetics and pharmaceuticals. In general, the type of products it refers to are topical products that contain ingredients that influence the biological function of the skin. However, the term can be misleading to consumers who may incorrectly believe that cosmeceuticals have the same strict rules and regulations for quality control and efficacy as pharmaceuticals. Cosmeceuticals are neither recognized by the U.S. Federal Food, Drug, and Cosmetics (FD&C) Act of 1938, nor are they regulated by the FDA.

Even for dermatologists and skin care professionals, regulations can get confusing and overwhelming at times. Whenever I return home from the American Academy of Dermatology's annual meeting, my luggage is filled with oodles of the newest and latest age-defying lotions and potions. At the 2010 annual meeting, "snail slime" was all the rage. I wanted to try it because I make it a point to sample everything and read all of the literature so that I can bring back only the very best new products to my practice.

It's important to help my patients separate fact from fiction when choosing cosmetic products that claim to significantly turn back the clock. I find it outrageous when I see advertisements on TV that promise consumers that their latest creams will mimic the effects of injectable fillers and lasers. For every new in-office cosmetic procedure that emerges in the world of cosmetics, it seems like there is a cream being announced that supposedly can achieve similar results in as little as seven days. These "hope in a bottle" remedies are usually just emollient creams that help hydrate the skin by preventing epidermal water loss and improve the appearance of fine wrinkles.

However, due to recent medical advancements in the aesthetic skin care industry, we have a better understanding of how the skin ages and which active ingredients work best to slow down the aging process, reverse the signs of sun damage, and protect the skin from future intrinsic and extrinsic aging. The challenge is to match the appropriate ingredients for a particular skin type or disease and to weed out ingredients that don't have any physiological effects on the skin.

This begs the following questions: What are the differences between the skin care products that are bought in a department store or pharmacy and those bought in a medical office? And furthermore, how do skin care professionals evaluate skin care products before offering them to their patients?

The main difference between over-the-counter skin care products found in department stores and those found in a doctor's office is that most dermatologists and skin care providers closely evaluate the active ingredients in a product and ask manufacturers for peer-reviewed evidence about the efficacy of the active ingredient of their products. They also ask for before-and-after photos and histological studies to ascertain if there has been a marked improvement in the quality of the treated skin.

When such high standards are applied to cosmeceuticals, it is easy to screen out products that do not show any substantial benefits in reversing the signs and symptoms of an aging skin. In other words, you won't find products with unsubstantiated claims in a competent dermatologist's office. The bottles you're offered may not look as sleek and beautiful as those found in a department store, but the active ingredient will have a significantly more beneficial physiological effect on the skin.

Companies will sometimes create two versions of their products: those that you can easily find in a department store and those that you can only get in a doctor's office. The difference is that the "MD" formulations have a higher concentration of the actual active ingredient. There is a direct correlation between the concentration of an active ingredient in a product and its effectiveness: the higher the concentration of the active ingredient, the better its efficacy. Once a dermatologist has determined that a particular product meets the criteria of safety, efficacy, and cost, the next step is to discern whether or not the product contains an adequate concentration of the active ingredient to have a physiological effect on the skin.

Finally, product stability is taken into account whenever a product is under the scrutiny of skin care professionals. While a particular product can start off with a sufficient concentration to have a meaningful effect on the skin, it can also degrade fairly quickly when exposed to light or air, causing it to lose its potency. If a product's potency and stability are in question, a dermatologist or skin care professional can request a high-performance liquid chromatography (HPLC) test from the manufacturer to assure that the product maintains its potency and stability over time. Most reputable skin care product manufacturers have the adequate instrumentation in their labs to conduct a HPLC stability study of their products.

This helpful tool allows dermatologists and other skin care

professionals to choose only those products for their patients that have an adequate concentration and stability of a particular active ingredient. There are many options out there, but if you stick with those products containing peer-reviewed evidence and ingredients that affect the skin's physiology in a positive way, your skin will be more radiant and reflect a much younger age.

In the next section, I will discuss proven cosmeceutical options for skin renewal, photoaging reversal, and skin nourishment and protection. I will start with the best key active ingredients, and then mention different treatment options for specific needs and skin types.

## RETINOIDS

Retinoic acids and derivatives are the most powerful topical treatments on the market to reverse the signs and symptoms of photoaging and to maintain the elasticity and integrity of the skin. All retinoids are derived from vitamin A, which is essential for normal growth, healthy bones, skin development, and the renewal of body tissue. A deficiency in vitamin A has been known to cause night blindness, acne lesions on the face, dry scalp, and the formation of thick skin plaques on bony prominences, such as knees, elbows, and heels.

The most effective treatment for the aforementioned conditions used to be eating foods rich in vitamin A, such as liver or cod liver oil. In the 1930s, the observation that skin conditions responded to foods rich in vitamin A led to the insight that using vitamin A on the skin could have curative properties for multiple skin conditions. Later, in the 1970s, new synthetic analogs and derivatives of vitamin A were introduced at full speed to treat common and more serious skin disorders.

By now, most of us are familiar with the trademarked ingredient, Retin-A. The generic name for this chemical is tretinoin (retinoic acid). The medical uses for the miraculous retinoid creams that incorporate tretinoin include most types of acne, psoriasis, and several other skin disorders. For the past few decades it has been the number one dermatologist-recommended age prevention and reversal cream worldwide.

Retinoids are extraordinarily effective in reversing the signs and symptoms of aging because they behave like hormones. They have gene receptors that, when activated, can reverse the signs of aging and photodamage. For example, when the retinoic acid receptors (RAR) or retinoic X receptors (RXR) are activated, they can prevent the activation of enzymes called matrix metalloproteinases (MMPs). These enzymes lead to the production of collagenase, which fully degrades skin collagen. In addition, these receptors also activate the production of new collagen and elastic fibers and hyaluronic acid.

Retinoids can greatly help to prevent the breakdown of the existing collagen and elastic fibers, and  to generate more of each. Retinoids may even prevent photodamage by inhibiting the induction of MMPs after one is exposed to UV radiation. It is necessary to stop using retinoids for at least five to seven days prior to sun exposure to avoid getting sunburn. Since retinoids increase photosensitivity, it is possible to become sunburned rather quickly when using them.

Another biological property of retinoids is their ability to act as antioxidants by scavenging free radicals. Free radical exposure comes from environmental and dietary sources, and it can cause cellular damage to the skin.

I am a big advocate of using retinoids. Since many patients abandon their treatments of retinoids because of too much discomfort, we start its use slowly. There is a potential for redness, itchiness, dryness, and photosensitivity while the skin is adapting. With patients who have never had any experience with retinoids, I usually start them with retinol. Later, they graduate to retinaldehyde (in other words, retinal), which is one step up from retinol. I call retinol and retinal "training wheels" for tretinoin. Once my patients are ready to graduate to the prescription-strength formulation, I start them with the lowest dosage and have them mix a pea-sized quantity with two pumps worth of my proprietary formulation, B-Sensitive™ lotion (Shino Bay Cosmetic Solutions).

B-Sensitive lotion is a calming moisturizer with natural anti-inflammatory properties that reduce the redness and drying sometimes associated with prescription retinoids. When patients are ready to move up in strength, I slowly increase their dosage.

*Caution:* Pregnant patients should stop using topical retinoids because of the potential of systemic absorption and the correlation of oral retinoids with birth defects.

*Caution:* To prevent adverse reactions with other treatments, I advise patients to stop using any retinoids a week before doing any laser procedures, chemical peels, microdermabrasion, or waxing.

It is very important for consumers to know that even though some products sold over the counter may claim to have retinol as their active ingredients, their concentration or stability may not be sufficient to have an impact on the skin. I recommend La Roche-Posay, SkinMedica, Neutrogena, and Roc® skin care lines. These are reputable, over-the-counter product lines containing retinol that are manufactured and packaged properly in order to ensure their efficacies.

After a patient has gotten used to the retinol cream, they can start to move up the ladder to retinaldehyde-containing products. The Avène® brand is sold at doctors' clinics and has a great formulation, retynal, which comes in various strengths. The Avène formulation, Diroséal, is perfect for those patients either with very sensitive skin or rosacea who would like to have the benefit of a retinoic acid.

There are several formulations of first-generation retinoic acid and its derivatives. My favorite ones are Retin-A Micro, Renova, Refissa, and generic tretinoin cream. They are all different prescription formulations of tretinoin. Some of them even contain an active ingredient that is slowly released into the skin to prevent irritation.

There are other formulations, such as Differin cream (adapalene), that are less irritating than the other retinoic acids but are still very effective. Once my patients have maxed out their benefits with all other retinoic acids, I usually graduate them to Tazorac (tazarotene) cream. It can be a lot more irritating than the other retinoids, so you have to work your way up to it. Nevertheless, it is an amazing product to reverse and improve severely photodamaged skin and wrinkles.

*Caution:* It is an absolute contraindication to use Tazorac while pregnant because tazarotene has a strong potential to cause birth defects.

## HYDROXY ACIDS

Hydroxy acids have been around for a long time. Everyone knows about Cleopatra's ultimate beauty secret of using sour milk on her face and taking milk baths in order to achieve a flawless complexion from head to toe. Was she out of her mind or is there actually some benefit to this beauty ritual? Sour milk contains lactic acid, an alpha hydroxy acid that penetrates the skin, causing the old skin to slough off and promoting the growth of new skin. Thus, I would imagine that she must have had the softest, freshest skin of her time!

Before anyone goes through the trouble to create their own lactic acid with sour milk, it may be helpful to know that there are many different forms of hydroxy acids that have similar molecules and functions. Hydroxy acids are organic carboxylic acids classified into alpha hydroxy acids (AHAs) and beta hydroxy acids (BHAs). Most AHAs are derived from natural sources like fruits and milk.

The AHAs most commonly used by the beauty industry are glycolic acid, citric acid, mandelic acid, and lactic acid. These acids serve to decrease the signs of aging by gradually lifting off the surface layer of dead, leathery skin cells to reveal a smooth, even-toned complexion underneath. In a nutshell, hydroxy acids are phenomenal skin retexturizers. In order for AHAs to be effective, their concentrations and pH need to be adequate. The optimum pH for them to work well with the natural pH of the skin is between pH 3 and pH 4.

The greater the concentration of hydroxy acid, the easier it is to unglue the layers of dead skin cells. Products containing a concentration of AHAs in the 5–10 percent range tend to be most effective. Concentrations higher than 10 percent are not allowed to be sold as over-the-counter products, but they can be utilized for in-office treatment in a medical clinic or skin care facility.

People with very sensitive skin may not be able to use AHAs because of possible itching, redness, and burning sensations. A milder alternative are the BHAs. The most commonly found beta hydroxy acid is salicylic acid, which is a mild, but effective skin exfoliator. Most over-the-counter salicylic acid products have a concentration no higher than 2 percent. Higher concentrations are used in doctors' offices as mild chemical peels, and these do wonders for acne-prone skin and for the elimination of blemishes.

AHAs and BHAs cause photosensitivity, so it is important to have adequate sun protection while you are using them and to stop using these products at least five to seven days prior to receiving any laser treatment.

In our practice, we have creams, pads, and lotions containing different formulations of glycolic acid and mandelic acid to help our patients retexturize their skin. My favorite lines are our proprietary formulation of 10 percent and 15 percent glycolic acid creams and pads (Shino Bay Cosmetic Solutions) and Vivite from Allergan. The Vivite line has a proprietary formulation with a slow-release glycolic acid that helps my patients to achieve a skin texture that is even and radiant.

NuCelle® is a wonderful product that I encountered while attending my first annual meeting of the American Academy of

Dermatology. After receiving a kit, I tried it with my usual skepticism. To my surprise, not only did my skin look visibly younger and more radiant, but it also helped stop my occasional breakouts. I started to sell it to the nurses at the hospital, and they saw great results, as well. In fact, I became so busy with this new venture that I eventually handed the operation over to a friend so that I could concentrate on my studies.

## ANTIOXIDANTS

It's important to separate fact from fiction when it comes to the antioxidant family. Although there are numerous topical antioxidants in the cosmetic industry, very few have peer-reviewed evidence about their physiological effects on the skin. Even the well-known vitamins C and E need to be in a certain form and contain a specific concentration to have a significant effect on the skin.

The role of antioxidants is to scavenge and neutralize the free radicals that bombard our skin and bodies every day. Free radicals are formed inside our bodies as a byproduct of our digestive processes. They are also formed by exposure to external factors, such as pollution, acid rain, and radiation—including the electromagnetic fields generated by our smartphones and other electronic equipment. Why should we worry about free radicals? As you'll recall from Chapter 3, free radicals are reactive oxygen molecules that have the capability of causing oxidative cellular damage to every cell in our body.

Free radicals are unstable molecules that have one unpaired electron. Since they are highly reactive due to this unpaired electron, they search for electrons in order to become stable molecules. Free radicals achieve their pairing of electrons by "stealing" electrons from surrounding molecules or cells. The excessive bombardment of free radicals on cellular membranes causes tissue damage. It is postulated that every cell in our body gets attacked by a free radical at least every ten seconds. When free radicals damage or mutate enough healthy cells in our bodies, the aging process begins.

There are enzymatic systems in the body that scavenge free radicals. But perhaps the best active strategy we can use against free radicals is to ingest foods—fruits and vegetables mainly—that terminate the chain reaction of the oxidative process on a chemical level. Our bodies don't manufacture these micronutrients, so they have to come from food or nutritional supplements. The main antioxidant micronutrients to look for are vitamin E, vitamin C, and beta-carotene.

The best way to illustrate the protective nature of antioxidants is by examining how the process of oxidation affects an apple. Within minutes of cutting into its bright red or green protective skin, it starts to turn brown and withers. What kept the apple fresh beforehand was its skin. Apple peel is rich with antioxidants, including polyphenols, vitamin C, and carotenes. Once the antioxidant-rich skin is peeled, the protective barrier is gone and the oxidation process immediately begins to cause the apple to age and rot. If you squeeze the juice of a fresh-cut lemon over the apple pulp, the pulp won't brown because of the vitamin C in the juice.

Antioxidants protect our bodies from free radical attack by giving up one of their own electrons to stabilize the free radicals roaming our bodies. Unlike free radicals, antioxidants do not become unstable when they lose an electron. Once the free radicals become stable, they no longer need to attack our cells; thus stabilizing free radicals prevents premature aging.

The role of antioxidants when applied to the skin has shown some surprising benefits in age prevention and age reversal. However, it is important to be aware that just because some new exotic fruit has achieved the title of "antioxidant of the year" does not mean that it has better antioxidant properties than its predecessors. The molecules can sometimes be too big or unstable to have a significant physiological effect on the skin.

## *VITAMIN C*

This delightful, water-soluble vitamin, besides being tasty in oranges and other citrus fruits, is also very important for the normal functioning of the human body, including the formation of collagen. A deficiency of vitamin C can lead to bruising, gum disease, premature aging, and scurvy. Since it cannot be synthesized by the human body, the ingestion of vitamin C (ascorbic acid) is essential for the human body.

In the past, sailors used to suffer from scurvy because they would go for months at sea without ingesting any fruits or vegetables. Corkscrew hairs would appear on their bodies, open wounds would fail to heal properly, and their teeth would become loose and fall out of their bleeding gums. Doctor James Lind, a Scottish surgeon in the British Royal Navy, proved in 1747 that scurvy could be prevented by eating citrus fruits. The sailors began carrying limes on their open-sea voyages. It was not until 1932, however, that vitamin C deficiency and scurvy were causally linked.

Vitamin C interferes with the formation of reactive oxygen species (in other words, free radicals) and serves to decrease inflammation and redness after sun exposure. Applied topically, vitamin C has been shown to improve fine to moderate wrinkles after only three months of use. Although the mechanism of action is not 100 percent understood, it is commonly known in laboratories that the addition of vitamin C to cultures of fibroblasts increases the production of collagen.

There is no doubt that vitamin C plays a starring role in the production and preservation of collagen in the skin; however, when applied to the skin, it needs to be in the form of L-ascorbic acid to have any real benefit, as the compound destabilizes and quickly becomes ineffective when exposed to light and air. Therefore, it is very important to use stable formulations of vitamin C. Studies show that the addition of vitamin E and ferulic acid may help stabilize vitamin C, thus maintaining its effectiveness when applied to the skin. The bottom line is this: Don't buy any creams that claim to have vitamin C without asking the right questions. It is very important that the right molecule of this vitamin is used and that it is supplied to you in a peer-reviewed formulation with proven stability. Only formulations that contain at least 10 percent ascorbic acid have been shown to have any cosmetic and clinical benefit when used with regularity.

The best vitamin C-containing products recommended in our practice are the clinical line of vitamin C serums, such as Pro-Heal Serum and Pro-Heal Serum Advance Plus (made by iS Clinical), SkinCeuticals products containing vitamins C and E and ferulic acid, and the Glytone antioxidant line, which contains a proprietary formula of time-released vitamins C and E and red tea.


## VITAMIN E

This vitamin is really a compound of eight naturally occurring molecules of tocopherols and tocotrienols, which collectively function as vitamin E. Only one of those eight, tocopherol is the form of vitamin E that has internal benefits in the human body when ingested. The other tocopherols and tocotrienols are only useful as topical antioxidants. Vitamin E is the major oil-soluble antioxidant in the plasma and cell membranes of the body. Its role is to stop the propagation of free radicals that attack and destroy cell membranes.

Although people have used topical vitamin E for years to improve the cosmetic outcome of scrapes, burns, and other types of skin wounds, there is little evidence that vitamin E leads to an improvement of injuries and surgical scars. Still, millions of people claim to have had an outstanding improvement of their scars after using vitamin E as a treatment.

Vitamin E has been used cosmetically for years to improve wrinkles. I remember my grandmother opening her little capsules of vitamin E and applying vitamin E oil around her eyes. Some people claim that it is also effective in preventing the emergence of cold sores and for soothing minor to moderate sunburns. In addition, topical vitamin E has been shown to prevent the formation of sunburned cells and to reduce the inflammatory response related to sunburns when applied prior to UV radiation.

Among the formulations containing vitamin E that are recommended in my practice are the antioxidant Glytone line, which contains time-released vitamins C and E plus red tea, and SkinCeuticals C E Ferulic (containing vitamins C and E, and ferulic acid). Even though it is not clear whether topical vitamin E has the amazing antiaging properties that we see with vitamin C, in combination they work synergistically to create the perfect topical antioxidant.

## *FERULIC ACID*

Although this phenol-derived antioxidant only came into the cosmetic world at the beginning of the twenty-first century, it has been studied for years in animals due to its effect on cancerous tumors. Ferulic acid has been shown to cause cancerous cells to "commit suicide" (in other words, to undergo apoptosis) in cases of breast and liver cancer.

Ferulic acid is found in nature in the seeds of various plants, such as pineapple, orange, coffee, and rice. It is a potent antioxidant that makes the cell walls of plants strong and rigid. Of the few products containing ferulic acid, we recommend the SkinCeuticals C E Ferulic®. The addition of ferulic acid to this serum activates the antioxidative properties of vitamin C and vitamin E and improves their chemical stability. Studies clearly show that the addition of ferulic acid to vitamin C and E increases the ability of the skin to protect itself from photoaging up to eight times more effectively than without it.

## *ALPHA LIPOIC ACID*

Although present in most foods, this naturally occurring anti-oxidant is found in higher concentrations in liver, spinach, and broccoli. First discovered in 1951 and identified as part of the famous Krebs cycle that we all had to memorize in Biology 101 in high school, it takes the role of a coenzyme and helps in the production of cellular energy. The antioxidative properties of this water-soluble and fat-soluble antioxidant were discovered when the signs and symptoms of vitamin C and vitamin E deficiency improved with its consumption.

One of the best and most unique properties of alpha lipoic acid is its ability to neutralize free radicals in fatty and watery regions of cells. Researchers in the late 1980s quickly realized that this was a very powerful and unique antioxidant. In addition, alpha lipoic acid tends to recycle other antioxidants, such as vitamins C and E, thereby increasing our armamentarium against free radicals.

While most of the benefits described above come mainly from the consumption of alpha lipoic acid, there is very little data on its effects when topically applied to the skin. In high concentrations or mixed with other antioxidants, I believe that it has some amazing free radical scavenging and photodamage-prevention abilities. The best formulations with high concentrations of topical alpha lipoic acid are those developed by Nicholas Perricone, M.D.

## *UBIQUINONE (CoQ10)*

This oil-soluble substance is better known as coenzymeQ10 (coQ10). A quinone derivative that is present in the mitochondria of cells, it is essential for the generation of energy in all living cells in the form of adenosine triphosphate, better known as ATP. It's estimated that 95 percent of the energy of the human body is generated during this aerobic cellular respiration process. Early in life, the human body is able to generate all of the coQ10 that it needs on its own; however, as the body starts to age (or due to some medications), the levels of coQ10 start to diminish. As a result, the cells in the body begin to lose their ability to withstand stress and free radical attacks. In fact, this enzyme is usually regarded as the most accurate biomarker of aging, since its levels decline significantly as we age.

The scientific community is especially interested in coQ10 for its ability to act as an antioxidant and for its beneficial effects on the cardiovascular system and in metabolic disorders. Some people with congestive heart failure, hypertension, or migraine headaches have found relief with coQ10 supplementation.

There is little data about the benefits of topical coQ10 on the skin. In theory, this substance can neutralize the free radicals that have been caused by environmental sources or were created during cellular respiration. The molecule of coQ10 is relatively small, so it readily penetrates the skin upon application. Studies have shown that following exposure to UVA radiation, ubiquinone can deactivate collagenase production, the enzyme that breaks down collagen in the dermis. Once considered the most powerful skin care antioxidant available, ubiquinone scored better than the five most popular antioxidants in its ability to neutralize free radicals.

## IDEBENONE

This product came out originally under the name of Prevage® and was introduced as the most powerful antioxidant on the market. As you might guess, I couldn't wait to try it. Unfortunately, the first batch that came out on the market caused me to break out horribly. This felt devastating because I really wanted to experience the effects of the most powerful antioxidant in the world. The company quickly found out about this little setback that customers were having and reformulated the product. The new formulation was perfect, and everyone, including me, has since tolerated this product very well.

Idebenone is a synthetic analog of coenzymeQ10. As it is 60 percent smaller than regular coQ10, it penetrates the skin more readily and delivers its antioxidative protection with greater efficacy. Another major difference is that idebenone works internally at the cellular level in the mitochondria. Created by a Japanese pharmaceutical company in 1986, idebenone opened up a new door in the field of molecular biology.

Studies conducted in Germany showed this bright orange powder's capability to prevent cellular damage and skin aging, opening the doors for research in many fields where cellular repair and regeneration were important. For example, studies in the field of neurodegenerative diseases, such as Alzheimer's disease and ataxias, have shown some promising results. Having a potent antioxidant that neutralizes free radicals and assists in cell regeneration is the magical potion that we've long awaited.

Free radicals that attack our cells to steal that missing electron arise from a multitude of environmental sources. They also arise from our own cellular energy production metabolism. Idebenone targets the mitochondria, which are the source of internal oxidative stress of the cell. Therefore, it does an outstanding job at scavenging and neutralizing the damaging free radicals that are produced in the process of cellular respiration.

When cells are constantly bombarded by free radicals, they remain in a constant state of inflammatory oxidative stress. This oxidative state inhibits their capacity to repair themselves. Idebenone, by neutralizing the free radicals, fosters an environment where cells can repair themselves and keep up their youth and vitality. If the cells in our bodies retain their youthfulness, this translates into youthful tissues and organs—in other words, a more youthful you!

Of the many formulations of idebenone out on the cosmetic market, Prevage MD has the highest concentration of this super-powerful antioxidant. The Prevage MD has 1 percent of the active ingredient, idebenone, which is 50 percent more than over-the-counter formulations.

## *POLYPHENOLS*

Polyphenols are plant-derived chemical substances that act as natural antioxidants. Abundant in nature, they are commonly found in green, red, and white tea leaves and in grapes, berries, pomegranate, soybeans, and red wine.

The benefits of polyphenols have been studied and researched for several decades. It is therefore safe to say that consuming fruits and vegetables containing these fascinating compounds, or taking polyphenol-rich supplements, will have a positive impact on your health and longevity. Polyphenols have shown some promising benefits in treating inflammatory conditions, lung disorders (for example, asthma), cardiovascular disorders (for example, hypertension), coronary artery disease, macular degeneration, and a variety of cancers.

Studies have shown that regular use of polyphenol-rich creams and lotions may provide protection against sun damage and oxidative stress. However, the bioavailability, stability, and concentration of the active ingredient must be adequate for the desired results.

There are a multitude of polyphenolic antioxidants that exist in the cosmetic industry. In this book, I will only discuss those polyphenolic antioxidant creams and lotions that have been proven to produce marked improvements in photoaged skin and are backed up with peer-reviewed data.

## GREEN TEA

Most mornings, I start my day with a tall green tea latte made using low-fat milk and no sugar. Green tea is an ancient beverage known for its energy stimulating and medicinal properties. Most of the medicinal and cosmetic benefits of green tea can be attributed to its polyphenolic compounds. The major polyphenolic constituent found in green tea is from a subtype called catechins.

When applied topically, catechins have been proven to be effective in reducing sun damage. The protective capability of green tea comes from its ability to neutralize free radicals and reduce inflammation. Additionally, studies have shown that skin treated with a topical green tea formulation shows less DNA damage after UV radiation.

Due to the anti-inflammatory properties of green tea, many skin care physicians use products rich with green tea to soothe sensitive skin, including skin with rosacea. In my practice, we recommend Replenix CF, a green tea-rich product from Topix Pharmaceuticals, Inc., that is 90 percent polyphenol, plus caffeine.

## COFFEEBERRY

According to recent studies, the pulp of the coffeeberry is loaded with more antioxidants than any other naturally derived antioxidant on the cosmetic market. The extraordinary benefits of the coffeeberry were first discovered by a simple observation of the hands of coffee farmers. Despite working in the scorching sun, the hands and lower arms of coffee handlers appear soft, smooth, and wrinkle free.

After studying the components of the coffeeberry, a group of scientists developed a patented coffeeberry (cascara buckthorn) extract that has shown promising results in decreasing fine lines and wrinkles, and in improving problems of pigmentation. According to the oxygen radical absorbance capacity

(ORAC) assay, it has ten times higher antioxidant activity than green tea, blueberries, cocoa, and pomegranate. This is a comparison assay that ranks existing topical antioxidants according to their ability to neutralize oxygen free radicals.

The benefits of topical caffeine go beyond cosmetics. Recent studies have demonstrated that topical caffeine can prevent the occurrence of skin cancer caused by UV radiation. Special staining techniques of cultured human skin cells demonstrated that coffeeberry extract was superior even to green tea extracts in preventing photodamage when used prior to being exposed to UVA radiation.

I therefore recommend coffeeberry extract to any of my patients who have severe skin sun damage or a history of precancerous or cancerous lesions. The coffeeberry extract products recommended in my practice are from CoffeeBerry® Natureceuticals™ (made by Priori) and Revaléskin Organoceutical. With a 1.5 percent coffeeberry extract, the Revaléskin has the highest concentration available on the market. It is a potent antioxidant that helps to minimize the formation of precancerous lesions. Anyone with severe sun damage should use a coffeeberry extract product as part of his or her skin care regimen.

## NIACINAMIDE

This water-soluble vitamin from the B3 group is also known as nicotinamide or nicotinic acid amide. The terms nicotinamide, niacin, and niacinamide are used interchangeably to refer to any members of this family. It is found in the body as the coenzyme nicotinamide adenine dinucleotide (NAD) and is involved in the metabolism of carbohydrates.

Niacin is a familiar name to most of us due to it being one of the most essential nutrients in the human diet. While in medical school, I learned about pellagra, a disease caused by a severe deficiency of niacin in the diet. Niacin deficiency is usually observed in areas where people eat corn as their staple food. Corn is the only grain that contains low amounts of niacin. The symptoms of pellagra are severe diarrhea, dementia, and dermatitis. Left untreated, it can have fatal consequences.

Niacin can also be used to lower cholesterol and other lipids. In addition, there have been some promising studies about niacin improving the symptoms of Alzheimer's disease, anxiety, and depression. When choosing a niacin oral formulation, be sure to purchase flushing free niacin. Otherwise you'll get hot flashes.

Whether taken orally or topically, niacinamide has been shown to be effective in mitigating a number of inflammatory skin conditions, such as rosacea, acne, and seborrhea. Many dermatologists therefore include it as part of their armamentarium to help alleviate inflammatory skin conditions. In addition, studies have shown that niacinamide has an antitumor effect on sun-damaged skin cells and suppresses carcinogens after UV radiation.

Other studies show the ability of topically-derived niacin products to improve the adverse effects of chronic sun exposure and to reduce the incidence of precancerous and cancerous skin lesions. Niacin is now considered an important factor in assisting the skin to protect and repair itself from sun damage and aging. I recommend Nia 24™ for people with severely sun-damaged skin.

## DIMETHYLAMINOETHANOL (DMAE)

This naturally occurring substance is a biochemical precursor of acetylcholine, a neurotransmitter responsible for muscle contraction that is found in sardines, salmon, and anchovies. In several studies, DMAE has been shown to improve the cognitive functioning of aging patients. It has also been shown to decrease lipofuscin and the molecular waste that is found in the neurons, skin, and heart tissue of older individuals. DMAE decreases the levels of lipofuscin by decreasing the crosslinking of proteins that create this molecular waste in aging cells. DMAE helps with skin-tightening and is beneficial in reducing the progression of sagging skin. From the several products containing DMAE on the market, I recommend the line of Dr. Perricone.

## PEPTIDES

Peptides are polymer chains formed by the linking of amino acids. If you recall from Biology 101, proteins are also formed by linking amino acids. The difference between a protein and a peptide is in their structural flexibility. Peptides are flexible chains of amino acids without one preferable conformation, while proteins maintain some preferable conformation. Peptides function as messengers carrying vital information and signals between cells and tissues. Basically, we could not function without peptides. Hormones, neuropeptides, antibiotics, and toxins are a few of the most important peptides that we are familiar with today.

The role of peptides in the skin is to keep the cells of the epidermis in communication with the cells and tissues of the dermis. This is extremely important for proper wound healing after an injury. As communication diminishes within the skin as part of the normal aging process, there is a decrease in collagen and elastic fiber production. This is also correlated with a decrease in the expression and function of key skin peptides.

One of the hottest peptides for skin rejuvenation that I came across during my residency was copper peptide. Not only was it great for wound healing, but it also functioned to reverse the effects of aging on the skin. Copper peptide is just that—a peptide tightly bound to a copper atom. Studies have shown that this particular peptide has the capability to reduce scar formation by inhibiting inflammation and the accumulation of large collagen aggregates that are typically seen in a scar. It also stimulates normal collagen production, helping the tissue on the scar to resemble the normal skin surrounding it.

Remember, when collagen is made slowly over time, instead of in a hurry, it resembles the collagen in healthy skin. In severely sun-damaged skin, we find aggregates of unwanted, broken-down collagen and elastic fibers (in other words, solar elastosis). Since we would like to stimulate new collagen and elastic fibers to replace the old, using copper peptides should, in theory, improve wrinkles.

In summary, copper peptides create a cascade of biochemical events under the skin that lead to skin remodeling. When purchasing peptide-containing copper products, it is important that an adequate concentration of the active ingredient is present and that there are no other ingredients in the cream that may interact with the ionic copper. If the ionic copper is neutralized, there will be little benefit; even worse, it could generate copper complexes that inhibit cell replication.

The bottom line is that you should only choose products that come from reputable companies that invest in research and quality control assays to ensure that there are enough stable copper peptides in their products. In my opinion, Neova® Copper Peptide Skin Therapy is the leading brand utilizing this technology. Many plastic surgeons recommend it to their patients for postoperative procedures to improve wound healing and to minimize scars.

There are a lot of new peptide-based creams on the cosmetic market with long, complex names and numbers. They are all working towards the same goal: stimulating new collagen and decreasing wrinkle formation. The most popular are those containing palmitoyl pentapeptide-3 (the 3 is sometimes changed to a 4, but it's basically the same molecule), also known as Matrixyl®. This peptide works at the DNA level to stimulate new collagen and fibronectin. Fibronectin is part of the cellular matrix of the skin and is important for cell adhesion, growth, migration, and communication. An increase of collagen and fibronectin leads to a healthier, younger-looking skin.

Dermaxyl® (palmitoyl oligopeptide) is one of the new peptides commonly used in skin care products. The main function of this peptide is to restructure the key components of youthful skin. Many studies have demonstrated this peptide's ability to help the skin generate its own collagen, elastin, and hyaluronic acid. When all of these elements are increased, you can expect to see a skin that looks smooth and rejuvenated with a better texture.

Matrixyl 3000 is basically Matrixyl (palmitoyl pentapeptide-3) plus palmitoyl tetrapeptide-7. Each ingredient has been shown to have distinct age reversal qualities at the molecular level. When palmitoyl tetrapeptide is added to a cultured human fibroblast, it stimulates it to lay down new collagen, hyaluronic acid, and elastin.

Argireline® is the trade name for another peptide, acetyl hexapeptide-3/8, which was developed by Lipotec, a company in Barcelona, Spain. This peptide works by limiting muscle contraction. It softens the muscles controlling facial expression, helping to relax the face and prevent wrinkles.

It is very important that products claiming to contain this peptide come from a reputable company with a sufficient amount of peptide (5–10 percent concentration) in a stable form. Having a proper concentration and stability are important criteria for a product to be able to deliver on the results that it promises. Just because a product package lists a certain active ingredient does not mean that it has the adequate concentration or capacity to achieve the same results as other products.

SNAP-8 is the trade name for acetyl glutamyl octapeptide-3. This molecule is simply an elongation of its predecessor, Argireline. It works by reducing the contraction of the muscles of facial expression, thus decreasing the depth and quantity of wrinkles, especially around the eyes and forehead.

There are many other products containing peptides available on the market. I tend to recommend only the products that I have personally tried, along with the ones that have produced great results with my patients. In my practice, we recommend Make Me Younger (Shino Bay Cosmetic Solutions), a peptide-rich moisturizer treatment, which contains Matrixyl and Dermaxyl; Replenix® AE Dermal Restructuring Therapy (Citrix); the C8 Peptide product line (Kinerase); Gentle Rejuvenation (Obagi); or Environ™.

## GROWTH FACTORS

Growth factors are naturally occurring substances that promote and support cellular growth and proliferation. Cytokines and hormones are two examples of growth factors. In reality, they are oligopeptides that act like signaling substances between cells. As their names imply, growth factors can be thought of as fertilizer for the skin. They act as messengers to stimulate collagen growth and to provide nourishment for skin cells. Growth factors can be derived from plants, animals, cultured epidermal cells, placental cells, and human stem cells.

Based on the growing demand of consumers for smarter and more effective cosmeceuticals, cosmetic companies are introducing a variety of recombinant growth factors in their formulations to aid in age prevention.

## HUMAN GROWTH FACTORS

Human growth factors are derived from human tissue, such as placenta, foreskin, and other cultured cells. Different types (in other words, families) of these growth factors have different jobs. The most commonly used human growth factors in cosmetics are transforming growth factor-beta (TGF-beta) for tissue regeneration, epidermal growth factor (EGF) for cell growth, and fibroblast growth factor (FGF) for wound healing.

My first experience with a human-derived, growth factor-rich cosmeceutical was with SkinMedica's TNS Recovery Complex®, one of the first products ever to use human growth factors. It sounded promising, and it was recommended by my attending physician for a patient during my residency. The patient was eager to try it until my attending physician told her that the product was derived from a baby's foreskin. After an initial look of repulsion crossed her face, she sighed and said, "Anything for beauty." Although the product's very distinct smell kept me thinking about its origins, it was cosmetically elegant, and I did see an improvement in some fine lines around my eye area after a few weeks of use.

I think the company worked on the smell because we didn't hear too many complaints after the first batch. TNS Recovery Complex uses a patented ingredient called Nouricel-MD™, which was, in fact, bioengineered from an original donor baby's foreskin. However, there is no reason to get grossed out. After the first extraction of growth factors from the cultured skin cells, all that was left were the amazing signaling oligopeptides that help transform your skin. TNS Recovery Complex contains TGF-beta, keratinocyte growth factor (KGF), vascular endothelial growth factor (VEGF), and hepatocyte growth factor (HGF). They all work synergistically to promote new collagen in the dermis, thicken the skin cell layers in the epidermis, repair photodamage, and decrease inflammation.

Another product that we recommend in my practice is the Neocutis with PSP® line. The simple observation that fetal skin has a unique ability to heal without scarring prompted Swiss medical researchers to compare and contrast normal wound healing in mature skin versus fetal skin. The data strongly suggested that the scarless wound healing of fetal skin was the result of a unique blend of growth factors and cytokines. Based on these impressive findings, a blend of human growth factors, cytokines (in other words, peptides), and interleukins (in other words, groups of peptides) was developed and used in multiple skin care and pediatric burn studies.

This miraculous concoction was labeled PSP for Processed

Skin Cell Proteins. The PSP complex contains TGF-Beta 3 and all of the other isoforms of TGF-Beta that are believed to be extremely important in the transition between scarless wound healing and repair scar formation. Other ingredients included in the mixture are basic fibroblast growth factor (bFGF), epidermal growth factor (EFG), keratinocyte growth factor (KFG), granu-locyte colony-stimulating factor (GCSF), insulin-like growth fac-tor (IGF), and vascular endothelial growth factor (VEGF). This naturally balanced blend of growth factors and cytokines has demonstrated in multiple studies that it has the capability to restore and rejuvenate aging skin in as little as two months of regular use.

## ANIMAL-DERIVED GROWTH FACTORS

Animal-derived growth factors have recently made their appear-ance in the world of cosmetics. Snail slime is the one causing all the rage at the moment. It sounds gross, but I have to admit that the product works wonders for the skin. For the past five years, I had seen advertising on Spanish television for different prod-ucts containing snail slime. I often wondered to myself, What's next . . . crocodile tears? I have to admit, though, that sometimes nature does know best.

The slime provides this little creature with a lot more than just a means to slide and crawl around. Studies have shown that snail secretion contains fibroblast growth factors that help the snail's skin repair itself after an injury or sun damage. This pow-erful bioactive secretion stimulates the production of the ele-ments necessary to assemble the extracellular matrix under the skin cells. This matrix provides the structure for collagen depo-sition, hyaluronic density, and elastin integrity, which translates into the regeneration of aging or damaged skin.

While on a trip to Medellin, Colombia, I saw a man who was surrounded by a group of curious bystanders. As I approached,

I saw that he was selling . . . snail slime! He had actually brought the snails with him and was putting on a show. Even if snail slime has some rejuvenative properties, I did not feel safe putting something on my face that had not been sterilized. After all, these little creatures might have had some weird bacteria that could eat my face off if I got infected. That being said, I was still intrigued by the miraculous claims that this gentleman was saying about his 100 percent natural snail slime.

A few months after my trip, I attended the American Academy of Dermatology's annual meeting, and to my surprise, there it was, the new breakthrough in age intervention: snail slime. Since I don't believe in coincidence, I went to the booth of the company promoting it to get more information and some samples. The product's name is Tensage® (Biopelle®, Ferndale Laboratories, Inc.), and it contains a proprietary formula with SCA Biorepair Technology.

The SCA is the slime secretion of *Cryptomphalus aspersa,* a species of brown garden snail that biochemically stimulates vital processes to repair and regenerate damaged tissue. According to studies, SCA Biorepair facilitates the proliferation of fibroblasts; induces the reconstruction of the skin's architecture by increasing collagen and elastin production; increases the amount of moisture on the skin by increasing the density of hyaluronic acid; and reduces inflammation on the skin. In fact, this product has been used for over twenty years in Europe to help alleviate radiodermatitis and chronic inflammation of the skin after radiation therapy for certain cancers.

Finally, this wonder product has entered the United States cosmetic market. I was so impressed with the results from the samples that I decided to carry it in our practice. All of our patients and staff now love the product and tell me that they cannot live without it.

## PLANT-DERIVED GROWTH FACTORS

Just like human- and animal-derived growth factors, plant-derived growth factors have made an impact in the cosmetic industry. The most commonly used plant-derived growth factors for age intervention are kinetin, zeatin, and pyratine-6. These plant-derived growth hormones, which come from a family known as cytokinins, promote cell growth and regeneration. Several studies indicate that these cytokinins have a positive effect on human skin fibroblasts.

Kinetin (N6-furfuryladenine) and zeatin keep the fibroblast healthy and active, causing it to continue to lay down new collagen and elastic fibers. Kinetin improves the overall appearance of the skin by reducing the number of fine lines and wrinkles and by increasing the moisture content of the skin. Zeatin also slows the aging process and improves other signs of aging, such as discoloration and roughness.

Pyratine-6 (furfuryl tetrahydropyranyladenine) is the new kid on the block in plant-derived cytokinins. It is created in a laboratory by fusing the naturally occurring kinetin with a tetrahydropyranyl molecule. This alteration of the kinetin molecule causes it to have a rapid onset of action and results in greater physiological changes on the skin than its predecessors, kinetin and zeatin. In fact, most patients claim to see results in as little as two weeks. Some of the reported skin improvements include a decrease in redness and roughness, a reduction in visible signs of sun damage, and an improvement of fine lines and wrinkles. In addition, pyratine-6 has the ability to neutralize harmful free radicals that contribute to the aging of normal and sun-damaged skin.

Two different head-to-head independent studies were performed—one by the University of California, Irvine, and one by a laboratory in Texas—to compare the efficacy of kinetin and pyratine-6. After eight weeks of treatment, the results were in favor of pyratine-6. There was a reported 86 percent improvement in skin roughness with pyratine-6 versus a 35 percent improvement with kinetin. There was also a 22 percent improvement in fine wrinkles with pyratine-6 versus a 2 percent improvement with kinetin.

The products recommended in our practice that contain kinetin and zeatin are from the Kinerase® and Obagi® Gentle Rejuvenation skin care lines. Both lines have the appropriate concentration of the active ingredients, plus other synergistic ingredients that help reverse and halt the aging process of the skin. They are excellent lines for mature skin.

Pyratine-6 is the most reputable line containing this active ingredient. It is great for patients who want a topical treatment to increase their collagen reserves without any irritation. It is especially useful for patients with intolerant skin, like those who have rosacea or adult acne.

## ANIMAL-DERIVED STEM CELLS

Our practice was one of the first in South Florida to add stem cell masks to our armamentarium of skin-rejuvenating solutions. Since it has a reputation for quickening the recovery process after aggressive procedures, I decided to test it against the most powerful laser in my practice: the SmartSkin $CO_2$. We used the stem cell mask right after the SmartSkin $CO_2$ microablative laser. Five days post procedure, all patients looked as if they were already on week two of the healing process. The skin also appeared younger and brighter after a few weeks. We achieved such impressive results that not only did we become the largest user of the stem cell mask in Florida, we also became a field research center for this magnificent product.

The stem cells in the mask are placenta-derived stem cells from sheep. Mammalian stem cells are far more effective in human tissue than plant-derived stem cells. Embryonic-derived stem cells are essentially identical to human stem cells and have the enzymatic capability to help regenerate and rejuvenate the skin. Embryonic stem cells are pluripotent, which means that they can turn into any other type of cells. They also express the "immortality gene," NANOG, which helps the cells divide and multiply indefinitely without losing their ability to differentiate. This is great news because it means there are no cells in the body that cannot be repaired or replaced. Old and weathered skin cells can be replaced with a new generation of skin cells to create a younger complexion.

The stem cell mask can be used after any skin rejuvenation procedure, including chemical peels, microdermabrasion, and ablative and nonablative photofacials. It can also be used as a stand-alone skin-rejuvenation mask. The mask should be used once a week for a total of three to four weeks for optimal results.

## PLANT-DERIVED STEM CELLS

Most plant stem cells used today in cosmetics come from apples, specifically from Uttwiler Spätlauber trees indigenous to northern Switzerland. The apples from these trees are well known for their ability to stay fresh long after they are fully grown. It was speculated that their ability to stay fresh was due to their high percentage of antioxidants; however, further research discovered that their ability to stay fresh is because of their phyto stem cells. Researchers believe that plant stem cells have the ability to regenerate and rejuvenate skin cells. The end result is a refreshed and younger looking skin.

Even though the use of plant-derived stem cells seems promising in the cosmetic industry, there is very little scientific research data that proves that they have a major physiological effect on human cells. Nevertheless, most people that have used products containing plant-derived stem cells are happy with the results.

## OXYGEN BIOTHERAPEUTICS, INC.

Many people know that oxygen is the most abundant and essential chemical element for sustaining life. Oxygen is essential in the production of collagen and elastic fibers and plays an important role in many other cellular metabolic functions in the skin. It would therefore seem reasonable that using a cosmeceutical with the capability of increasing levels of oxygen in the skin would lead to impressive regenerative and rejuvenating effects. However, I was worried about products that claim to have oxygenating capabilities because they often use chemical activators, such as hydrogen peroxides, which dry out the skin. They also have the potential to generate unstable free radicals that can be harmful to skin cells.

At last, a new and innovative oxygen carrier serum concentrate and eye cream has been developed that can provide the skin with abundant levels of oxygen. Dermacyte® (Oxygen Biotherapeutics) is a state-of-the-art technology that helps transport pure oxygen into skin cells and surrounding tissue. This skin care line utilizes a patented oxygen carrier oxycite technology that is identical to one used to treat spinal cord injuries and promote wound healing. Studies have shown an overall improvement in skin tone and texture, and a decrease in fine lines and blemishes after as little as two weeks of regular use. Now there is even an amazing makeup line, Oxygenetix®, which we can use to camouflage the skin after having a laser treatment or chemical peel.

## ANTI-GLYCATION TECHNOLOGY

Glycation is a process in which sugars latch on to proteins, such as collagen and elastic fibers, creating crosslinks between them and causing the skin to become stiff and brittle. Glycation generates 3-deoxyglucosone (3DG), which impairs the ability of collagen and elastic fibers to function normally. The body is unable to break it down or to replace it with healthy new collagen, leading to a severe thinning and wrinkling of the skin. In addition, 3DG causes inflammation and the formation of free radicals that can assault and damage healthy cells. The older we get and the more sugar we consume in our diets, the more our skin and other tissues are negatively affected by glycation.

The damaging effects of glycation in human tissue are nothing new to the medical community. We have learned much about this phenomenon from researching diabetic patients. Most of the adverse complications seen in patients with diabetes are the result of the formation of advanced glycation end products, especially 3DG. Nerve damage, blindness, kidney failure, and diabetic skin ulcers are some of the most common complications observed in diabetic patients with advanced diseases.

There are two great products that counteract the damaging effects of glycation in the skin. MEG 21 with Supplamine® (Dynamis Skin Science) is a groundbreaking treatment discovered by the Dynamis Diabetes Research Team at Fox Chase Research Center. The scientists there were able to generate a compound that lowers the levels of 3DG in tissues. To their surprise, they saw an absolute rejuvenation on the skin, which actually makes sense since diabetics have greater amounts of 3DG in their skin. MEG 21 with Supplamine is a complete skin care line that has been clinically demonstrated to reduce the appearance of fine lines and wrinkles, as well as to improve the overall tone and texture of aging skin.

The other skin care line with ingredients that help block the glycation process is A.G.E. Interrupter by SkinCeuticals. This line contains a specific compound extracted from blueberries that interrupts the formation of advanced glycation end products (in other words AGEs).

## IONIC TECHNOLOGY

Does ionic technology sound like science fiction? Like laser light technology, perhaps? It is no secret that ions play an important role in the human body. In fact, without the proper flow of ions, the bioelectrical force that keeps us alive would be compromised, and we would cease to exist! Our metabolism depends on the body's bioelectrical energy to acquire nutrients and excrete waste. We also depend on it for muscle mechanics and locomotion, heart rhythm, and cell-to-cell communication.

It is well understood that as the body ages, there is a significant decrease in ionic flow, resulting in a decrease in cell-to-cell communication and collagen production. Diminished collagen in the skin leads to fine lines, wrinkles, and sagging skin.

Like any other organ in the body, the skin cells take advantage of this bioelectrical force to communicate important messages among themselves. The scientists at Neutrogena who were aware of this intricate phenomenon developed the Neutrogena Clinical line with Ion Complex technology. This breakthrough in skin care increases the positive ions flowing within the skin's surface, thereby helping to maintain the ongoing creation of new collagen and preventing the breakdown of the skin matrix.

The product comes in a package with two little tubes. The first tube contains a dark gray gel that has a proprietary formula with essential ion-mineral conductors; the second tube contains an activating white cream. When the tubes are combined, it causes a positively charged ion flow within the skin's surface. The end result is a more resilient, hydrated, and toned skin that looks and feels younger. After trying this product for myself, I was definitely pleased and impressed with it. I have since recommended it to all of my patients.

## PUTTING THE INFORMATION INTO PRACTICE

After reading about different products and the science behind them, I am guessing that you might be feeling a little lost or unsure of how to use the information. Allow me to break it down. During the day, we need to protect our skin from free radicals, the environment, and the sun. At night, when the body and soul rejuvenate, it is important to use products that are designed to repair and regenerate skin cells and to replenish the matrix of the skin. I encourage all my patients to use some kind of retinoic acid. You can also add a moisturizer or treatment that contains peptides or growth factors to your nighttime routine.

I advise my patients to rotate their use of products. The skin can get a little lazy when a certain product is used continuously over a long period of time. For example, I often switch the family of retinoic acids that I use at night. I use tretinoin for a few months and later switch to tazarotene, and vice versa. I do the same thing with my antioxidants, peptide creams, and growth factors.

I started to alternate my use of products after observing that patients who had been using the strongest dosage of tretinoin for years had maxed out on the benefits of this wonderful product. When I switched them to another family of retinoic acid, they started to see some improvement almost immediately. After all, if you always do what you've always done, you'll always get what you've always gotten! So don't be afraid to experiment or try new things. You never know! You just may find the holy grail of topical skin rejuvenation.

The future of skin care is looking better than we have ever dreamed possible. Understanding the skin at the molecular level of genomic technology has opened up an unimaginable world. It has helped us to identify important biomarkers of skin aging and has allowed us to create smarter skin care products that can intervene in the aging process. Genomic research for the treatment of aging skin is still in its early days, but it is paving the way for a new generation of skin care products that will make everything that has come before it obsolete.

It is important to be aware of the ingredients and the mechanism of action of all products that you use, as well as to keep in mind the intention of why you are using them. When I apply a particular eye cream, for example, I envision that every cell in my body is listening to my intention. So, when applying your own products, tell your cells to start generating new collagen and elastic fibers to rejuvenate your skin.

# CHAPTER 11

# Beauty Is Where You Find It

---

Several years ago, I was at the Atlanta airport waiting for my connection home to Florida when something happened that would change the course of my practice forever. I had finally achieved my dream of becoming a cosmetic dermatologist. I had the office of my dreams. I had been invited to be one of the main speakers for a Cynosure lasers conference. Yet something was bothering me. I wasn't happy with myself. My job, which usually gave me joy, had become a bit of a drag. I felt depressed and didn't understand why.

While I was waiting for the plane to start boarding, a book with a shiny silver cover caught my eye. It was practically calling out to me, so I got up to see what it was about. The book was *The Power of Impossible Thinking* by Yoram R. Wind. Since I tend to read spiritual and self-help books, I decided to purchase it. As I was reading it in the airport, I saw a drawing that I had once seen in a psychology class during college. It was the famous perceptual illusion of the "beauty" and the "hag," a cartoon entitled "My Wife and My Mother-in-Law" by W.E. Hill published in 1915 in *Puck* humor magazine. Depending on how you look at it, your brain switches from seeing the image of a young, beautiful woman or an ugly, old woman.

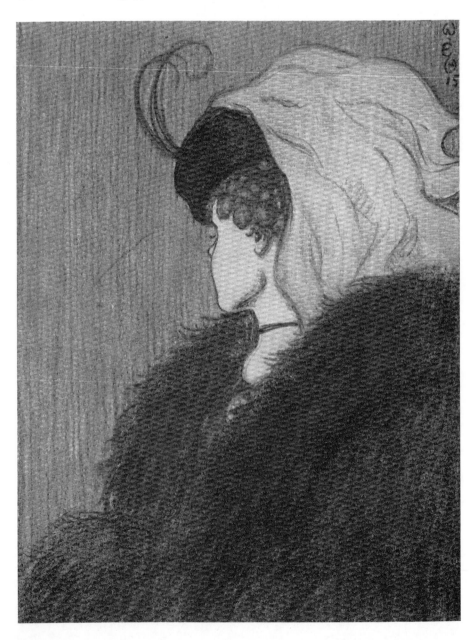

No matter how hard I tried, all I could see was the old woman with the hooked nose. It was extremely frustrating. The previous time I had seen the drawing I'd been able to see both figures in the drawing in a matter of seconds. It then became clear what was really wrong with me. During my training as a resident, and every day thereafter as a cosmetic dermatologist, I was either looking for imperfections to correct on people's faces or people were coming to me to show me their imperfections. Thus, I had become conditioned *only* to see people's imperfections. I had stopped seeing the beauty in people. No wonder I was sad. This realization felt like a tremendous awakening, and it gave me the opportunity to see life in a different light.

Ever since that experience in the airport, I strive to see the beauty in everyone and in everything around me. Now, when people come in for a consultation, I always first look for the beautiful features in their faces. We all have them—some people may have more than others, but everyone has beautiful attributes. When using fillers and Botox, I strive to bring symmetry to the face, replenish facial volume loss, and restore the youthful contours of the face. However, first and foremost, I always focus on accentuating the attractive attributes that are already present on someone's face.

We've already learned that beauty is a precise phenomenon based on the laws of mathematics. It is an evolutionary advantage, and today more than ever we feel the pressure to stay young. We are constantly bombarded with pictures of beautiful models and actresses accompanying advertorial articles in magazines. We even have television programs about extreme makeovers that turn "ugly ducklings" into "beautiful swans."

On the quest to stay young and beautiful, many people have sacrificed the humanity of their faces. They may have fewer wrinkles and tighter skin after being treated with surgery or injections, but they often look bizarre—and sometimes even inappropriate. I've learned a lot about human behavior and the psychology of beauty since I began to dedicate 95 percent of my practice to aesthetic treatments. And it's important to understand that although beauty may have a formulaic basis, the perception of beauty fluctuates according to decade, ethnicity, and individual preference.

## SEXUAL DIMORPHISM

By definition, sexual dimorphism is the difference in form between males and females. These differences determine what the opposite sex considers attractive in a potential mate and varies by race, time period, culture, and location. There are a few features, however, that are universally accepted as hallmarks of attractiveness for males and females. Women usually find a prominent chin, strong brow, and a square jawline attractive in men. Women also find a distinct body shape attractive in men: tall, with a slim waist, muscular chest, and broad shoulders. We can add having washboard abs and a minimal amount of body hair to the list.

For their part, men find women with large eyes, a small chin, a petite nose, full lips, clear skin, and high cheekbones attractive. Men are also more attracted to women with specific body proportions—these tend to vary a bit from culture to culture. In the United States and in other parts of the Americas, men prefer women who are slender (but not too skinny), full breasted, and have hourglass figures.

There is a scientific explanation as to why some characteristics cause the opposite sex to find a person attractive. The universal male and female secondary sexual characteristics mentioned above are signs of apparent genetic and reproductive fitness. The more of these characteristics a person has, the more attractive he or she will be to members of the opposite sex.

All of the aforementioned attractive features are the result of developmental events that are under the control of sex hormones during puberty. Estrogen, for example, is thought to make the bottom part of a female face narrower and the cheek-bones wide and rounder.

After menopause, and with the decline of estrogen, a woman's skin becomes thinner, drier, and starts to wrinkle. In addition, the lips become thinner, the eyes smaller, and the cheeks start to drop. These changes all signify a loss of youthfulness and reproductive capacity.

By comparison, testosterone in males is responsible for the square jaw, strong brow, and thick upper bridge of the nose. With age, men experience andropause, during which the decline of the hormones testosterone and dehydroepiandrosterone begin their decline. While andropause does not cause a man's reproductive system to stop working completely, it may lead to bouts of impotence. The decrease of testosterone also leads to an accumulation of mid-body fat and the loss of musculature and youthful characteristics.

Testosterone-dependent secondary sexual characteristics signal immunological competence, strength, and survival abilities, all of which were important traits to protect and provide for a family in a more primitive era. As human beings evolved, good looks became more important to a female than a man's fighting and survival abilities. Facial symmetry and beauty advertise better genetic material and health.

Recently, several studies have concluded that facial features that are more characteristically feminine are more attractive for both men and women. These studies show that feminized male faces are more attractive than the average masculine face. The so-called pretty boy male tends to do better with the ladies than the average masculine Joe after puberty. The process of natural selection has changed quite a bit since the Stone Age. According to some psychologists, women are attracted to males with feminine features because they associate them with other desirable characteristics, such as parental ability, honesty, loyalty, and cooperation.

It is important not to mistake an effeminate face for a face that has feminine facial features mixed with secondary male characteristics. Only Mother Nature is able to achieve this combination without making a man look bizarre. Whenever I am doing fillers on a man, I make sure to use a different technique than what I customarily use for a woman. If I were to use the same technique, it would carry the risk of feminizing my client's face and making him look really weird. This is also the reason why a full facelift hardly ever looks good on a man: Most of the face lifting techniques cosmetic surgeons use tend to feminize the face.

Continuing with the subject of looking peculiar, we have all encountered people in our daily lives (or perhaps on TV) that just look, for lack of a better word, unnatural. I live near the Boca Raton area in Florida where I see a lot of women wearing the same face—just on a different body. When new patients come to see me for a consultation, they often tell me straight away that they don't want to have the "Boca babe" look. It's funny because I know exactly what they're referring to. It also reassures me that I am not hallucinating when I see the same face everywhere.

I'm not sure if this is a new trend—like the Angelina Jolie lips were a few years ago—or if it is a reflection of where we are going with aesthetics. Do these people look in the mirror and say, "Wow, I look gorgeous!" or do they say, "Oh my God, I really went overboard with this"? I am getting more and more convinced that they truly believe that they look great.

From time to time, some of these people have consultations with me. They come in with extremely over-filled cheeks, Spock-like eyebrows, and lips that enter the room before they do. I am thinking that they probably want some sort of laser treatment or some skin care advice, but no—they want more fillers and more Botox! Although it is a hard thing for me to do, I have to turn them down. I don't want to hurt anyone's feelings, so I try to be as kind as possible. I tell them that as a minimalist I am not good at achieving that particular look.

They appreciate the honesty and usually don't return because I'm not a good match for them as a cosmetic dermatologist. That is my point! The patient's perception of beauty has to match the perception of beauty of the doctor.

I tell all new patients from the beginning that I don't believe in frozen faces or overinflated cheeks and lips. If they are in agreement, then we're a good match. If they feel, however, that I am too conservative in my approach, then they can go to someone who can give them the look they want.

During consultations, I educate my potential patients about the aging face and what they can do in each decade to help prevent its descent and deflation. I also encourage them to seek consultations with other cosmetic dermatologists so they can choose the doctor who best understands their needs and matches their perception of beauty. One piece of advice is to notice the look of the staff and other patients in the reception area. Also, be sure to ask to look at before and after pictures of patients. This will help you determine whether the doctor's perception of beauty matches your own.

Even though people with overinflated cheeks and frozen faces may look unnatural to me, this is only *my* opinion and *my* perception of beauty. If these patients truly feel younger and more beautiful, who am I to make them feel otherwise?

Every year, I go to the American Academy of Dermatology's annual meeting to take some courses and see what's new in the aesthetics world. The sixty-eighth meeting was held in Miami Beach in March 2010. I was surprised to see a few of my friends and colleagues with the Boca babe look. I thought to myself, *It's become an epidemic!* However, I finally figured it out. Ever since we discovered that fat volume in the face is one of the key ingredients of the fountain of youth, we have been trying desperately to replace the volume loss. In the process, however, have we not lost sight of what it means to preserve the human attributes of a face?

I came back from my meeting and told my staff, friends, and patients to shoot me if I ever go that overboard with a cosmetic procedure. If I hadn't had the experience of the beauty and the hag at the airport, perhaps I would have become an adult Cabbage Patch Kid myself. I have to admit that I was once very close to looking like one. I was looking a little gaunt and tired so one of my friends injected some filler in my cheeks. I ended up looking like a marionette! I had such round, feminine-looking cheeks that I could barely look at myself in the mirror for nine months while the filler lasted. Fillers should be used in such a way that it's not obvious to everyone that a procedure has been done.

Today, anyone can look and feel beautiful. Cosmetic procedure advancements have opened up a world of opportunities for people who, genetically speaking, were not born with the blessing of perfect ratios and proportions. All it takes are financial resources and a capable surgeon with a keen eye. We've all seen the incredible transformations on TV shows like *The Swan* and *Extreme Makeovers*. Right in front of our eyes, we can see an ugly duckling transform into a beautiful swan. We've all also witnessed the powerful impact these changes had on the subject's persona.

It is my personal and professional experience that the better you look, the better you feel—so long as you have a healthy self-esteem.

One thing that I learned early on in this industry is that I will never be able to please everyone. I've met many patients who are never truly happy with the way they look, no matter how much improvement they see in their physical appearances. Having such low self-esteem, they will always find another flaw.

I even have patients who literally come to me with pictures of magazine models and ask me to give them a particular model's jawline, nose, cheeks, or eyes. Ironically, their natural noses, eyes, or jawlines are often ten times more beautiful than the model that they aspire to look like. These are red flags that tell me that I am probably dealing with someone with a poor self-image and low self-esteem. It breaks my heart because I know how difficult and all-consuming it is to feel that way.

A dear patient of mine wrote me a letter of gratitude that

truly illustrates how a small procedure that lasts only twenty minutes can help someone with a poor self-image feel better. He elected to have facial fillers and a microablative $CO_2$ laser resurfacing of the skin and had outstanding results. This is an excerpt from the letter he wrote.

> *Dear Dr. Shino,*
>
> *I can't thank you enough for what you have done for me. As you know, I have body dysmorphic disorder (BDD). As I have aged, I have become very concerned about my facial and bodily appearance. Even as a young child, I never felt good about my-self. I persevered and became well-educated, which elevated my self-esteem. I can't believe that I look this good, and I owe it to you. Thank you, Dr. Shino. God is your partner, and he watches over you and wants you to continue changing people's lives.*
>
> *Sincerely,*
>
> *M*

I was very touched by this letter. Here is my brief response back.

> *Dear M,*
>
> *Your letter was very touching and put tears in my eyes. You probably don't know this, and very few people do, but I also suffer from a touch of BDD. I have struggled with it since childhood, and although I can write a whole book on the subject, I have made peace with the fact that what I see in the mirror is not the way I actually look or how people see me. I understand this disease quite well. It has also made me more sensitive and compas-*

*sionate, with a greater understanding about the little things that may cause someone to seek my expertise. I have since learned to look beyond the imperfections to see the beautiful attributes that we all possess. BDD was my curse, but it is also my blessing. It has forced me to see true beauty everywhere and in everyone.*
    *God bless you.*
    *Shino*

BDD comes in different grades. While some people, such as myself, have just a touch of it, many suffer from a more severe case. Individuals with this disorder are excessively preoccupied by a perceived defect in their physical appearances. They are usually considered very attractive to other people, but are unable to see this for themselves. It is a debilitating disease that results in a fear of judgment, social anxiety, low self-esteem, and obsessive-compulsive behaviors.

The exact cause of the disease is still debated, but most physicians believe that it could be a combination of psychological, biological, and environmental factors. In many cases, abuse and neglect have been primary contributing factors. These patients can be a cosmetic dermatologist's or plastic surgeon's nightmare. They are impossible to please and are always looking to alter the way they look. Nevertheless, you don't have to suffer from BDD in order to have self-esteem issues or a poor self-image.

My touch of BDD can be tracked all the way back to my early childhood. While hearing two of my aunts conversing, I overheard one of them telling the other, "Poor Shino—he is so dark and ugly." I was only seven years old, but right then and there I became convinced that I was too dark. I began to hate my skin tone. My cousins and the other relatives of my generation either looked Chinese or had lighter skin. I wanted so badly to have a lighter complexion that I even bathed in Clorox bleach to get my skin to turn lighter. My aunt's words made me feel that being dark equated to being ugly, so I spent the rest of my childhood and adolescence staying away from the sun.

Another reason for my touch of BDD is that I've always been what you might call, a "pretty boy." The times when my hair was a little long when I was growing up people would ask my grand-mother if I was a boy or a girl. My grandmother therefore made sure to get me crew cuts so that people knew that I was a boy. Due to my feminine features, I was beaten up by other boys in my elementary school pretty much every day for three years. I hated the way I looked, and I couldn't do anything about it. In my head, I was born deformed—as a boy who looked like a girl.

When Madonna came out with the song, "What It Feels Like for a Girl," it brought me back to those days when my life was hell because of the way I looked. It was okay for a girl to look like a boy, but for a boy to look like a girl was a reason for constant punishment and ridicule. To this day, when people come and see me they often use words like *pretty* or *beautiful* to describe me. Instead of making me feel good, I often feel embarrassed and uncomfortable by this. Men can be *handsome* or even *cute,* but *beautiful* is a term that you would use to describe a woman.

It is very important for parents and caregivers to be aware of the potential impact that their words can have on children. Neg-ative comments can cause a child to have a preoccupation with body image and cause emotional wounds that linger for the rest of the child's life. Not all of us are going to inherit genes that make us look skinny or beautiful, but we can all have a healthy self-esteem and positive body image.

I am well aware that my job as a cosmetic dermatologist is about much more than just slowing down the darn clock or re-versing the aging process. Whenever I am doing a laser proce-dure or treating someone with an injectable, I am also infusing a healthy dose of love and acceptance. When my patients look in the mirror, I want them to celebrate the essence of who they are. It is an emotional facelift as much as a physical one.

In my quest to bring a state of well-being to my patients, I spend my free time reading books about spirituality and self-help. I found a great book written in the 1960s by Maxwell Maltz, M.D., a renowned plastic surgeon. Considered by many to be the foundation of many of the self-help books that exist today, *Psycho-Cybernetics* teaches a practical way of living that ensures a life of happiness and fulfillment by using the power of the subconscious mind.

The most useful chapter in Maltz's book for me is the one entitled, "How to Give Yourself an Emotional Facelift." Some emotional scars need to be treated with a spiritual scalpel. My patients often come to me with their insecurities and fears. Some of them may be going through a divorce, some are petrified about the aging process and some of them may have a disfiguring scar from a surgery or an accident. No matter their initial reasons for coming in, however, they all have one thing in common: They want to be more physically attractive.

With my help, my client's fears and insecurities might just disappear. Although everyone has some degree of fear or insecurity, I discovered fairly quickly that I can only really help those patients who already have a relatively healthy self-image. It takes an enormous amount of time and effort to help patients who do not. No matter how great the improvements that I make for them, these kinds of patients are rarely happy for long.

Study after study has shown that beautiful people are treated differently. We tend to view attractive people as more honest, trustworthy, and intelligent than less attractive people. Since we are living in a society where fashion, cosmetics, and fitness are multibillion-dollar global industries, there is a great emphasis on physical appearance. Those who are perceived as attractive are valued more in our world in many contexts than those who are not.

Being beautiful may be something that we may all want, but it can also be a double-edged sword. People who are considered beautiful also experience negative judgment and pain because of it. Very good-looking people often evoke jealousy from others or doubt that they are valuable for other reasons. I experienced some of this growing up, and during the time I was working as a runway model. As a child, I would get teased and beat up because of my looks. After puberty, when my secondary sexual characteristics started to take form, I became the guy that other guys wanted as a wingman because girls were paying me a lot of attention.

Nowadays, I can walk into a room and experience rejection and admiration all at once. People may find me attractive, question my sexuality, ridicule me, praise me, dislike me, or love me. From time to time it causes me anxiety, but it is easier to cope with now that I understand human nature and the science of beauty.

Another drawback of being good looking is that it may cause an inability to maintain long-term relationships. I've observed this particularly among my female friends who are extremely beautiful. They are used to being adored by so many men that it is difficult for them to choose one and settle down. As the years start to pass and their youth and beauty fade, they can find themselves feeling anxious and lonely.

Whether or not you were lucky enough to have been born with the great genes that produce a symmetrical face, one thing is certain: If you don't have the right personality and demeanor, your outer appearance won't compensate for your lack of inner beauty. Although we all initially tend to gravitate towards and appreciate beautiful people, if they have ugly personalities we tend to run for the hills. As Oscar Wilde wrote: "It's beauty that captures your attention; personality which captures your heart." Ironically, in the midst of writing this chapter, I had the opportunity to meet a beautiful young lady who soon thereafter became infamous as the "Beauty Bandit." Twenty-nine years old and very attractive, she came into my clinic for some aesthetic procedures. When it came time to pay for the services, she took off. Fortunately (for us), we have security cameras, and the police were able to use these images to arrest her later for grand theft. It seems that whenever her beauty treatments would need a touchup, this woman would pull the same stunt in another cosmetic center in town.

The Beauty Bandit became the poster child for the epidemic of women who are doing just about everything possible to preserve their beautiful attributes—even risking going to jail. While working on her, I distinctly remember that her eyes appeared dead. We kept staring at each other's eyes as if our souls knew that something bad was about to happen. After it was all said and done and the media had created a spectacle of her, I could only feel deep sadness for her and her parents. She was one of the lucky ones with great genetics and beautiful attributes, but she had chosen to use her attributes to live a life of chaos and darkness.

Years ago, a patient once had told me, "Beauty is wasted on the young." I could finally comprehend that statement. A beauty magazine contacted me and asked me if I could come up with a quote that would define my feelings towards the Beauty Bandit. I said, "Beauty is a double-edged sword that may cause you to experience both admiration and disappointment. The Beauty Bandit is a vivid example of this."

During my residency in dermatology, I already knew that my calling was to become a cosmetic dermatologist. My personal trials and tribulations were preparing me to have the skills and temperament necessary to enter the world of cosmetics. I was also aware that it was my duty to go beyond the realm of physical beauty. I feel that the spiritual purpose of my work is to help remove emotional scars and enhance people's self-esteem, and to teach the true meaning of beauty to everyone that I encounter.

Upon entering our clinic, our patients are greeted by a large poster of Audrey Hepburn with a powerful message by humorist Sam Levenson that is often referred to as "Time-tested Beauty Tips." Written for Levenson's grandchildren, these lines, which combine two passages from Levenson's 1973 book *In One Era and Out the Other,* just so happened to be some of Audrey's most beloved. When asked in an interview to share some beauty tips with her adoring fans, Audrey saw an opportunity to convey the true meaning of beauty. She recited Mr. Levenson's words:

*For attractive lips, speak words of kindness.*
*For lovely eyes, seek out the good in people.*
*For a slim figure, share your food with the hungry.*
*For beautiful hair, let a child run their fingers through it once a day.*
*For poise, walk with the knowledge that you never walk alone.*

*People, more than things, have to be restored, renewed, revived, reclaimed and redeemed; never throw out anyone.*
*Remember, if you ever need a helping hand, you will find one at the end of each of your arms.*
*As you grow older, you will discover that you have two hands: one for helping yourself and the other for helping others.*

These passages were sent to me by a friend on Monday, November 25, 2002, in an email bearing the subject line: "Beauty Secrets from Audrey Hepburn." Since the day I read them, I knew that this message, along with Audrey Hepburn's beautiful photograph, was going to be the focal point and message of our clinic. I wanted everyone to be reminded of what it truly means to be beautiful. Time-tested beauty starts from within, and those who practice being beautiful find it.

# CHAPTER 12

# Color Me Perfect

I can still remember my stepmother, Frances, getting up super early in the morning to do her makeup. It would take her almost an hour, and it was a Zen-like ritual for her. Every stroke of her brush was precise. Watching her was like watching an artist painting on a canvas. To this day, she is still a very beautiful woman, but as a younger woman there was not a single soul who wasn't enamored with her beauty when she was made up.

I have always wondered about the origins of makeup. Why do women draw black lines under their eyes? Why do the lips need to be red? Why do the cheeks need to be flushed and the eyelashes made to look like little tarantulas? There is even a Spanish adage that says, "If a lady is naturally pretty, she is beautiful. If she isn't, then she should be wearing makeup."

The ritual of makeup spans at least 6,000 years of human history, starting with the Egyptians around the fourth century B.C.E. Although perhaps not the very first people to wear makeup, the Egyptians were among the first to document using makeup to enhance their beauty. When we think of Cleopatra, we think of her black-lined eyes. Men and women made their eyes more alluring by using kohl, a substance made from metallic elements, such as antimony, lead, mercury, and copper, as well as from burned almonds and soot. Unaware of the danger of using mercury and lead as cosmetics, these Egyptians were literally dying to be gorgeous.

Ancient Egyptians, Greeks, and Romans alike used cosmetics to enhance physical appearance. In fact, archaeologists from every other continent also have documented the utilization of makeup for beautification. Even in the most remote areas of the world, aborigines have utilized natural dyes as paint to adorn their bodies.

Since its inception, makeup has been used to flaunt or disguise aspects of appearance. For example, during the Middle Ages and Renaissance in Europe, having pale skin was considered a sign of wealth thought to emphasize gentility and femininity. Some women would bleed themselves to the point of anemia in order to achieve the palest possible skin tone. They also used white lead paint, arsenic, and mercury powders to mimic fair skin.

A bizarre incident involving cosmetics took place during the Renaissance period in Naples. It revolves around the introduction of Acqua Tofana facial powder, named after its creator, the infamous Giulia Tofana, who is perhaps the greatest poisoner of all time. Containing a highly toxic arsenic liquid compound concocted by Signora Tofana and her daughter for sale to would-be murderers, the white powder, which was purportedly being used to achieve much-desired pale skin, was sold to wealthy women who were usually well aware that the product contained an extremely dangerous poison. Women were advised to dust the powder on their faces, necks, and chests—but only when their husbands were around.

You can imagine the outcome. There are over 600 known victims who died from being poisoned. Most of the victims were the husbands of unhappy wives, but some wives accidentally killed their husbands because they unwittingly used the facial powder for its advertised cosmetic purpose. Twenty years passed before Signora Tofana was arrested (and subsequently strangled in prison) for her crimes.

When the French introduced red makeup for cheeks and lips around the eighteenth century, having pale skin became associated with poor health and fragility. The use of heavy makeup or rouge became a way for many women to hide their illnesses.

Interestingly, men used makeup until the 1850s. Following that, it was frowned upon for a man to wear any kind of makeup on his face because it was considered too "dandy."

Early in the nineteenth century, during the Victorian era in England, the desire for pale skin returned. Having suntanned skin signified that someone had to work outdoors to earn a living. Therefore tanned skin was considered inferior, vulgar, and not "lady like." Women carried parasols to protect their skin from the sun in an attempt to remain pale. Wearing rouge or makeup became frowned upon in "respectable" society due to their association with stage actresses and prostitutes. During this period, the only cosmetic practice that was tolerated was to use hot wax beads mixed with egg whites as mascara for eyelashes. This glossy mixture was also used as pomade for the lips. Since rouge was no longer tolerated, women would secretly use beet juice or pinch their cheeks to obtain a healthy red glow on their faces.

The pale Victorian look dominated until the 1920s, when American women, in order to show off their individuality, started to embrace red lipstick, mascara, eyeliner, and face powders. Women began to paint their eyelids with different tones of gray. Colors like green and turquoise also became fashionable. Brow pencils and eyebrow tweezers were introduced, as most women preferred thin eyebrows with a downward slope. In addition to bringing women the vote and introducing less restrictive clothing with higher hemlines, this era inaugurated a makeup revolution. Women enjoyed an increased selection of colors and higher quality, safer ingredients in their cosmetic products. There was a marked shift in social attitudes toward makeup globally. It was no longer taboo to find beauty products in a woman's purse or to see women applying pressed powder or lipstick at the dinner table.

Another change in the perception of beauty occurred in 1923 when influential French fashion designer, Coco Chanel, was spotted with a deep, dark tan after yachting from Paris to Cannes. *Voila!* Having a tan suddenly became a fashion trend. A majority of the working class now had pale skin from spending most of their time working indoors in factories, so having a tan became a sign of leisure that demonstrated financial security, rather than the physical strength of a laborer. To this day, we still see the rich and famous spending their holidays basking in exclusive resorts or playing on their private beaches and yachts. Almost everybody loves to bathe in the sun by a pool or the ocean, though, unlike Chanel, we are slathered with SPF lotions when we do.

A lot has changed since the 1930s. We are constantly bombarded with new makeups and styles of fashion. Hollywood starlets have been setting trends in the world of makeup for decades. Who can forget Sofia Loren's unique cat eyes or Rita Hayworth's famous red lips, which were voted "most perfect" in the world by the Artists' League of America in 1949? In our era, iconic celebrities like Halle Berry, Jennifer Lopez, and Angelina Jolie influence women around the world to strive for certain looks through haircuts, diets, and fitness regimens, clothing, makeup, or via cosmetic enhancement procedures. Angelina Jolie was single-handedly responsible for the demand for full lips that we saw in the past several years, gaining her the adoration of many dermatologists and plastic surgeons due to the revenue that she brought into their practices.

Lipstick, eyeliner, and rouge are more than the apotheosis of good grooming for women. There is a lot of science behind the art of makeup. Most cosmetic companies employ a team of chemists and engineers who research, create, and test hundreds of new formulas a year. A lot of trial and error experimentation takes place until the right textures and shades are obtained. The final products need to be effective, elegantly packaged, and have pleasing aromas.

Scientists ensure that each and every ingredient of any cosmetic product is disclosed and that strict safety guidelines are followed in manufacturing the makeup. Before any cosmetic company can sell its products, it needs to put these formulations through rigorous trials to see how they weather varying environmental conditions, such as high altitude, humidity, heat, and cold. Finally, before being released into the marketplace, the product is tested on humans or animals to check for possible allergic reactions and to ensure that a makeup, skin lotion, or hair conditioner works according to its design.

Many companies no longer use animals for the testing of cosmetics, because forcing helpless creatures to endure the painful side effects of testing is cruel, and these companies usually announce this fact on their labels.

Besides helping us to conceal our flaws and accentuate our best features, makeup also helps us to feel confident, happier, and more attractive. No one likes to feel frumpy and dull at a social event. Makeup allows us to put our best faces forward, creating a feeling of elation that is interrelated with our brain chemistry. A physiological response tells us, "I look good, therefore I feel good."

Makeup also causes a physiological response in those who perceive the artistry. It creates the illusion that its wearers are younger, healthier, or more attractive than we actually are. For instance, using a foundation that conceals flaws in our skin tone advertises to others that we are seemingly fertile and disease free.

Using colored lipsticks has been in vogue off and on in the millennia of history recorded before the ages of either Cleopatra or Queen Elizabeth I. The fascination with full red lips has to do with only one thing: seduction. As blood shunts to the lips during sexual intercourse, the lips get larger and turn redder. Using lipstick triggers the physiological response of attraction because seeing plump red lips reminds us of the gratification that we experience during sex. It's perceived as an invitation.

Darkening the upper eyelid works in a similar way. During the last stage of sexual orgasm, the upper eyelid drops minimally as a physiological reaction to satisfaction. The "smoky eyes" or "bedroom eyes" makeup technique therefore makes women look like they are on the verge of having an orgasm, and produces an almost hypnotic effect on men.

As we age, our eyes become smaller and squinty. Drawing a dark line under the lower eyelid causes the eyes to look larger and wider. Therefore, using this simple makeup trick is another strategy to advertise youthfulness and to increase the perception that we are, in fact, attractive.

There are many makeup tricks to help us conceal our flaws, balance facial asymmetries and accentuate our best features. I have met many women who without makeup are not nearly as attractive as when they are made up. This evidences how a few strokes of a brush can turn someone's face into an enchanting work of art.

We have finally realized the art and science of making someone look and feel glamorous using makeup. Still, there are many considerations to be aware of when selecting a cosmetic, including the consideration of selecting a color that matches your skin tone and having a flawless finish that seems age appropriate. Unfortunately, I constantly witness women walking around looking ashy, ill, or like they're wearing facemasks. They have no idea that they're using the wrong foundation.

I dabbled in the art of makeup in my younger years while doing special effects for haunted houses and theatrical playhouses. I was great at turning someone into an alien or a zombie, but I could never make someone look more attractive in the way that a makeup artist can. I've therefore asked Loren Psaltis, a professional makeup artist, to share tips with us. A native of South Africa and one of my dear friends, she has agreed to reveal secrets for bringing beauty and balance to your face at any age.

# Makeup Advice for Any Age

## ADVICE FROM LOREN PSALTIS

The beauty of makeup! The only true instant-result procedure, makeup can be used to enhance and transform the face, or create illusions, or to conceal problems and flaws. Although there are many tricks, and only a few rules to applying it, correct makeup—in its truest role—simply makes the best of whatever you have in the most natural way.

The art of makeup belongs to everyone. You don't have to be a professional makeup artist to create professional looks. After all, who in the world knows your face better than you? Who else knows what feels comfortable and natural? Become your own expert and create a signature style that can be adapted for any occasion.

Our goal is to help you make correct product choices for your appearance and to learn proper makeup application skills. The best advice we can offer you is to invest some time experimenting in a department store, pharmacy, or cosmetic store to better understand the differences between the textures and performances of the various products that are available. With as many choices as we've got these days, finding the right makeup can be a confusing, expensive, and frustrating process, especially when the product we've chosen does not perform to our expectations. By adhering to the guidelines I'm about to give you, you can sidestep issues and create your best look.

I strongly advise you to sample before you buy. Products look and feel differently after a few hours of wear than they did upon first application. Also, since color is never accurately represented in department store lighting, you never want to purchase a product until you have tested it outside. Foundation, in particular, is best applied in natural light. If it looks great under natural daylight, it will look great under any conditions.

All reputable cosmetic companies provide sampling options. If you are looking at buying from a brand that only comes in sealed packaging, take along a little plastic container or a pill case so that you can take some home with you and test it first. Never buy a product without using it for at least a couple of days to ensure its performance.

For most women, realizing that they've been using the wrong kind of makeup is like discovering that they've been wearing the wrong bra size. It's a great relief! Makeup should be simple to apply, comfortable to wear. It should conceal our flaws and highlight our best features.

Although there are few rules, there are certainly some tried-and-true techniques that are proven to give great results. As with fashion, also always feel free to express yourself by experimenting with new trends and seasonal looks. Once you've developed a unique formula that suits you, a signature look, go ahead and make adaptations to update your look as needed from then on. It's important to take skin tone, age, occasion, personality, eye color, hair color, time constraints, and your profession into consideration when creating your look.

Your day-to-day makeup routine should take no longer than twenty minutes. Set this time aside each day for solitude. Put on some of your favorite music, relax, and focus on your thoughts. The phrase "Putting on your face" is an appropriate one as how you look has a big impact on how you feel. Applying makeup can become a personal ritual that sets the tone and mood for your entire day. Learn to enjoy this empowering feminine routine.

## GREAT MAKEUP STARTS WITH GREAT SKIN

Before applying makeup, your skin should be thoroughly cleansed. Residual oils from night creams that accumulate during sleep need to be removed before applying daytime treatments. Whether your preference is for a wash-off cleanser or a tissue-off cleanser, it is a good idea to follow up with toning. Toners remove residual cleanser and surface oils from the skin.

If your cleansing routine cannot be maintained, such as when you're traveling or at the end of the workday and going out right from the office, cleansing towelettes are a good option. They come in a variety of formulations ranging from exfoliating microbeads to super-soft lotions for sensitive skin. Conveniently, they combine cleansing and toning into one step—and they are extremely portable. Keep a couple in your handbag.

After cleansing and toning, apply eye cream and moisturizers. Allow these to be thoroughly absorbed into the skin before makeup application.

If you are using additional products, such as specialized serums, these should be applied before using moisturizer and should be followed by independent sun-protection products. Many moisturizers already contain sun protection.

The rule is this: When layering liquid products, ensure that you allow each to properly absorb into your skin before applying the next.

## TOOLS OF THE TRADE

Every artist or craftsman would acknowledge the importance of having the right tools for the task. Makeup artists are continually adding to their arsenals of brushes, sponges, eyelash curlers, and other accessories. Here are the ones I recommend.

## *BRUSHES*

You've probably seen makeup artists in specialty stores wearing military-looking pouches on their belts that are full of various sizes and shapes of brushes. That's because most people in the makeup business are a little obsessed with finding the perfect brush for a particular task. We've learned that the right brush can make all the difference in creating a perfect line, contour, or highlight, and for concealing a blemish.

Brush hairs, whether natural or synthetic, can make a huge difference in how much of a product or a color pigment a brush is able to hold. Spills of eye shadow onto a perfectly concealed under-eye area are traumatic! Brushes therefore should have an appropriate density and shape, as well as enough individual bristles, to allow the product to adhere. Although expensive, great brushes are a great investment since they can last for years with proper care. A good brush set is not going to shed and lose bristles and fibers.

Cheaper brushes tend to suffer hair loss at their bases, causing their densities to be quickly lost when the volume at their bases begins to thin. It can be frustrating to have to remove fallen brush hairs from your face and eyes constantly.

I prefer to buy individual brushes based on exactly what I need rather than a full set of brushes that may never get entirely used. Generally speaking, you need the following brushes. A brush for your:

- Powder.
- Concealer.
- Contour.
- Eyeliner.
- Bronzer.
- Blush.
- Base shadow.
- Highlighter.
- Lips.

Many makeup artists choose to apply foundation with a brush. Personally, I've never used a foundation brush on myself or any of my clients. I prefer finger blending it and sometimes using sponges to absorb excess product or to add it to other areas. This is a purely personal preference. If you are comfortable applying foundation with a brush, continue to do so and add it to the list of brushes you need above. Now, we will look at the specifics of each brush, including how to use each most effectively.

**Powder brushes** should be full, rounded, and soft. This last application of product to your makeup sets the look. The density of the brush is important. Blotches of powder on your foundation are difficult to disperse even with blending. Too much powder in one area can create a matte patch that makes the skin appear dull. Thus, the brush head should be so dense with fibers that it almost appears solid. A highly dense brush allows it to pick up an even amount of product. It is also important to remove any excess product from your brush by tapping off the loose product before lightly dusting it over your face.

**Blusher brushes** are smaller version of powder brushes. The circumference of the brush head is slightly more tapered at the outer edges. In contrast to the full roundness of the powder brush, it has a crescent-shaped dome. Blusher brushes collect less of the product than a powder brush and should lie flatter against the skin during application.

**Concealer brushes** are shaped for precise application. The head of the brush should have the appearance of a well-manicured fingernail with flat bristles and a soft oval crescent.

**Base shadow brushes** are used for the first application of neutral or nude shadow on the eyelid before color is applied. One of these should be a smaller version of the blusher brush shape.

**Contour brushes** are for use in the crease of the lid and therefore have a full, round soft bristle and specific tapering. As is the case with the powder brush and the blusher brush, the metal base of a contour brush should be round to allow for full dispersion of the bristles. The length of the bristles is important in a contour brush: The shorter the bristles, the harder the brush. Longer bristles allow for flexibility and smooth sweeping movements into the lid crease.

**Highlighter brushes** are for use under the eyebrow and into the arch of the brow. Their shape is similar to that of concealer brushes.

Personally, I use two **eyeliner brushes:** a very precise, small-pointed brush for liquid liner and a flat, horizontally precise, cut-edge brush for powder shadow. Both types of brushes should have a firm density of bristles because a lot of flexibility in the brush head can create an untidy line.

The horizontally edged brush has a thin row of bristles that only allow a small amount of shadow to be collected onto the brush. When working with dark eyeliner colors, we want to be especially careful to avoid an excess of powder particles from falling onto the under eye area and creating smudges.

**Lip brushes** should be firm, oval in shape, and dense. Since they are often used for blending two or more lip colors together, it is important to have a high enough density to hold a large amount of pigment.

**Bronzer brushes** should be the largest in your collection. Their loose density and super-soft flexibility are well suited for collecting a minimal amount of product onto the brush for a light application. Bronzer brushes may be used over the entire face, neck, and décolleté area.

Unruly brows need taming with a firm-bristled **eyebrow brush.** There are various techniques for shaping brows with color, including using pencil, powder, or liquid formulas. Whichever formulation you prefer, all tend to leave residue within the brow hairs. The eyebrow brush is effective for removing excess product, such as this, after shaping.

## *EYELASH CURLER*

An eyelash curler is invaluable for creating a wide-eyed look. Straight lashes do not create the illusion of framing the eye as well as curved lashes. Through experience, I've found that inexpensive brands are just as effective as the more upscale brands.

## *LASH SEPARATOR*

A fine-toothed metal comb with sharp points that are closely situated is necessary for separating lashes and removing clumps of mascara. Although many mascara brands claim to be clump free, I've yet to find one that doesn't clump, especially after the second coat. After each use, make sure to pinch the ends of the comb with a tissue to remove excess mascara from the comb. This is one implement that can get really clogged with product.

## *SPONGES*

Makeup sponges are versatile and come in a variety of shapes: rounded, squared, and wedged. They can be used for foundation and concealer application, for blending, and for cleaning away smudges.

## *TWEEZERS*

A good pair of tweezers is vital for shaping eyebrows, removing peach fuzz from your skin, and for collecting stray lashes, brow hairs, and any brush hairs that have fallen onto the face during makeup application. I have a collection of tweezers with various pointed and slanted edges for different uses. These are precision tools.

Since the engineering of the points makes a huge difference in their performance, investing in quality tweezers is wise. I only use tweezers made out of stainless steel. Cheaper metal alloys do not retain their sharpness, and painted finishes crack with time.

## PRIMERS, FOUNDATION, CONCEALERS, AND POWDERS

Regardless of the type of makeup you use—cream or liquid foundation, mineral powder, or tinted moisturizer—a foundation primer is essential for a flawless application. It also makes the foundation last longer. Primer should be applied after the full absorption of treatment products and should dry or set thoroughly before applying foundation.

There are many different types of foundation primer. Although they essentially perform the same function, their textures vary from brand to brand. The ideal primer should feel light to the touch, glide onto the skin smoothly, reduce the appearances of pores, and create the illusion of an even skin texture.

Most primers are colorless or skin toned. Their consistencies depend on their formulations and certain ingredients that act as line and pore fillers (for example, silicone). Ideally, primers should mattify the skin regardless of your skin type because foundation gives the final finish. When a primer is used in place of foundation to even out skin tone or correct textural problems, a specific formulation is required.

A primer with a dense viscosity is recommended for skin with large pores, and a rose-tinted primer adds warmth for sallow complexions.

For redness of the skin caused by inflammation, green- and yellow-based primers are great to cancel out red and purple. Dullness or a grayish hue can benefit from either rose tints or from radiance promoting primers that contain light reflecting particles.

Foundation is one of the most remarkable products ever developed to generate the look of great skin. It can also be the most frustrating of all products to choose correctly and apply properly. It is definitely a most rewarding discovery when you find the perfect foundation for your skin.

The most important factor when choosing foundation is how well it matches your skin tone. The only way to ensure that foundation is the right color for you is to test it in natural daylight. Department store and pharmacy lighting can be misleading. To reiterate, always take a little container with you to the makeup counter so you can ask for a sample of the tester. Take that home with you so that you can test the color against your skin in the daylight. Foundation must be tested on your face, not on your hand or arm.

I am surprised to hear that many makeup consultants test foundation on the wrist or the back of the hand. Apply the test color on your chin and forehead and then blend. A perfect match is when the foundation completely disappears against your own skin tone. An important consideration when selecting foundation is whether or not to match the neck skin tone. Many women have a pink hue in their faces that is not carried through to their necks. Ensure that the color you choose matches your neck tone. After application there should be no distinguishing lines between your jawline and your neck.

So how does that work? How can we choose a color that blends with the facial skin tone and the neckline if there is a difference between the two? First, foundation is primarily for the rectification of facial tone. The neck is naturally lighter than the face since it has less exposure to the sun. The chest, which is often more exposed to sunlight due to feminine necklines, is often darker than the neck in tone.

The foundation should match the face and blend seamlessly onto and under the jawline, which is always in natural shadow. Blending well at the jawline will prevent that telltale foundation line. We are not looking to match the face to the neck if there is a marked difference in tone; we want to make the face appear flawless and simply blend the defining application line between the two areas so that it is invisible. Powders and bronzers are convenient for evening out the color difference between these two areas.

Since the purpose of foundation is to correct uneven skin tone, the color should completely blend with your natural skin. Many women incorrectly choose foundation with the intention of creating a skin tone. They select hues with pink for warmth, brown for a tanned look, and yellow or ivory to cover redness. These issues are best dealt with, however, by using color-correcting primers, blush, and bronzers. Foundation's one and only job is to create a flawless—even natural—canvas.

The second most important consideration is texture. Foundation should feel comfortable and weightless on your skin regardless of the desired coverage. Even heavy coverage foundations and powders are available in lightweight formulations with adjustable concealing properties.

Choosing the right type of texture—the texture of a liquid, a cream, or a powder—depends on your desired look and comfort preference. It is also dependent on skin type. Very oily skin, for example, doesn't do well with creamy foundations. Dry skin may not be well suited for certain powder formulations. Coverage is also a factor. Tinted moisturizers generally do not conceal imperfections as well as more heavily textured creams or denser powder formulations.

Mineral powders can be a great option. They generally suit most skin types, are comfortable to wear, and allow adjustable coverage application more easily than some cream or liquid formulations.

Seasons of the year can also affect the choice of foundation. During the summer, you may prefer using a tinted moisturizer rather than a cream foundation, as warmer weather tends to negatively impact the staying power of creamy formulas. The oily T-zone area of the face (the forehead, nose, and mouth region) is particularly prone to shine as the day wears on. No matter which type of foundation you prefer, the most important consideration is how well it blends.

Make sure that the product you choose to apply is carried past the jawline if you are using it over the entire face. If you are using foundation only under the eyes or around the nose, blend well at the outer perimeter of the application area.

Skin type is a general guideline for choosing the formulation best suited for you. Here is a list of textures and the different types of skin for which they are formulated.

## *TINTED MOISTURIZER*

*Skin type:* Normal to dry
*Texture:* Lightweight cream
*Coverage:* Minimal
*Tip:* When using a tinted moisturizer, more coverage is needed under the eye area and for blemishes. Make sure to use a concealer over the product. If you apply concealer first, it will be removed by the creamy texture of the tinted moisturizer. Also, if you feel like you want heavier coverage on occasion, but do not want to switch to a foundation, concealer mixed with a tinted moisturizer will do the trick.

## *LIQUID FOUNDATION*

*Skin type:* All
*Texture:* Creamy liquid
*Coverage:* Light, medium, or heavy
*Tip:* Most liquid foundations are suitable to layer for adjustable coverage due to their light, liquid, creamy textures. Simply allow the first application to set completely (or blot the excess with a tissue) and apply another layer until the desired coverage is achieved. Also, feel free to mix foundations. I have found great success not only by mix-

ing different colors, but also by mixing different textures.

During the summer months when you have a tan, for example, you may want a lighter formulation than your regular foundation. Mixing a tinted moisturizer that's a couple of shades darker than your regular foundation into the foundation can create a lightweight version that matches your skin tone. During the winter months, when you may be a little paler and want more moisture in your foundation, mixing your basic formula with a moisturized formula that's a couple of shades lighter in tone should meet your needs.

## CREAM FOUNDATION

*Skin type:* Normal to dry
*Texture:* Firm, smooth cream
*Coverage:* Heavy
*Tip:* Cream foundation is versatile. It can be mixed with moisturizer to make it more of a liquid, or it can double up as a concealer when using lighter formulations. Cream foundation can also be made sheerer by applying it sparingly with a damp sponge. Using fingertip application gives the fullest coverage.

## STICK FOUNDATION

*Skin type:* Normal to dry
*Texture:* Solid cream
*Coverage:* Full
*Tip:* Although stick foundation is not the most popular formulation, commercially, it has a loyal following amongst those who prefer heavier coverage. It is also a great alternative to concealer and a good eyelid primer.

## MOUSSE FOUNDATION

*Skin type:* All
*Texture:* Whipped cream
*Coverage:* Medium
*Tip:* This is my favorite choice for mature skin because of its great absorbency. It doesn't sit on the skin like liquid or cream foundation do, and therefore it does not settle into lines.

## CREAM POWDER FOUNDATION

*Skin type:* Normal to oily
*Texture:* Solid cream (dries to a powder finish)
*Coverage:* Medium to heavy
*Tip:* It's a good choice for oily skin types since the powder properties absorb oil and counteract shine.

## MINERAL POWDER

*Skin type:* All
*Texture:* Loose powder
*Coverage:* Light, medium, or heavy
*Tip:* Mineral powders are wonderful because of their versatility. By using a concealer brush and a layering technique, you can fully cover blemishes, rosacea, and under-eye circles. Use a full round brush to get a light dusting of powder that will provide the least coverage. Also, by using a dense round brush and pressing into the skin in a circular motion, you can create heavier coverage.

## BB CREAM FOUNDATION

*Skin type:* All
*Texture:* Creamy
*Coverage:* Light
*Tip:* This formulation is the newest multitasking foundation available, boasting treatment benefits, primer properties, sun protection, and variable coverage. Although these new BB creams promise to do it all, I still use concealer under the eyes and add mineral powder for sun protection.

Concealers are indispensable in creating a flawless face. Beyond covering up dark under-eye circles and blemishes, they are wonderful for evening out the color of the eyelid and for preparing the eye for shadow. Concealers are also useful for contouring in shades that are darker or lighter than the base foundation color.

Powders are great for setting your makeup. They are also wonderful when you want to skip foundation and just even out your skin tone. They come in many shades, including translucent, and work with any foundation color to mattify and set makeup. Colored powders add tone to foundation. There are also powders with different degrees of shimmer that can be used in the evening or as bronzers.

Oily complexions should avoid using shimmer powders.

Powders come in a variety of textures, including loose or compact. Powders that come in a compact of mosaic pressed powder are good for sallow or red complexions when they include color-corrective pigments. The application of powder depends on the type of powder being used. Loose powders are applied with large, soft-bristled brushes and are gently dusted over the entire face. Compact powders are typically used with a puff applicator and are pressed gently onto the face.

## BLUSH AND CONTOURING

Blush has traditionally been used to add color and warmth to the face. Youth and vitality have always been associated with rosy cheeks. However, the application of blush has evolved into a more subtle use of color. The correct technique of contouring can create the illusion of an altered face shape. To add warmth to the complexion, add blusher to the apple of the cheek. To find the correct place to apply the color, simply smile and apply directly on the most prominent, fleshy part of the cheek. Then, sweep the brush up to the hairline along the cheekbone.

As far as color is concerned, it is a good idea to have two or three shades to complement different eye shadow and lipstick options: coral for reds, oranges, and yellows; pink for blues, wine, and mauve; and a nude to tan for natural or bronzed colors and for contouring. Used over the entire lid with a concentrated application, blush also doubles up as a quick eye shadow to create a natural, coordinated look.

Blush is more than the addition of color. It is one of the most effective and transformational tools for contouring the face. Contouring allows us to create the illusion of depth, shadow, and highlight. Using a darker shade of blush in the hollow of the cheek can create the illusion of a more prominent cheekbone and add a more sculpted look to a round-shaped face. To create a narrowing effect on a wide or square-shaped face, use the same contour technique and run the brush from the temples and past the earlobes down the sides of the face.

Although an angular or oval-shaped face rarely needs contouring, by applying the blush a little wider than normal you can encompass the hollow below the cheekbone and soften shadows. The rule of contouring is to use darker shades to create shadows and lighter shades to create highlights. Highlighting the orbital bone above the cheekbone gives a little lift to any face shape. This technique is most often used for evening or special occasion looks.

At all costs avoid very shimmery highlighters, as they most often look unnatural.

A long chin can be made to appear shorter by applying a darker blush color directly under the chin to create a shadow. A wide jawline can be narrowed in the same way by applying darker blush along the jawline, from the widest point to the earlobe. You can make a broad nose appear slimmer with subtle shading down the sides. The trick here is blending. The objective is to create natural looking shadows—not obvious lines.

For the purposes of contouring only, an absolutely matte, natural shade of blush should be used that is just a few shades darker than your foundation color. Another great option for contouring is to use a darker shade of mineral powder foundation.

## ALL ABOUT THE EYES

The eyes are the most important feature of the face. They convey our mood, show when we are weary, betray our age, and express our joy and excitement. Love is discovered through the eyes! We therefore need to make sure that we take great care of them. Eye makeup can be sultry and dramatic or natural and soft. Some dark eyeliner on the top and bottom lid at the lash line, and an extra layer of mascara, can change the most natural eye makeup into a dramatic, sexy look.

To create perfect eye makeup you need to begin with a perfect canvas. Preferably, use a concealer with a matte formulation to cover the top eyelid. Whether you're using a cream or powdered form, matte, oil-free concealers result in longer wear for eye shadow. Due to the thinness of the eyelids, many of us have red or slightly discolored lids where the underlying veins and capillaries show through. Using a concealer that acts as an eye shadow base is therefore essential. After preparing the lid, a nude color is applied over the entire lid.

Now is the time to study the shape of your eye. No matter the eye shape, the distance between the eyes, the lid space between lash and brow or the slant of the eye, there are techniques to enhance and transform any kind of eye. Regardless of eye shape or the look you are trying to create, by simply using two colors, a highlighter and a contour color, you can make up any look.

For the purposes of this chapter, we are discussing the best basic looks to suit any age. You will therefore be shown how to create your signature look for your everyday life. However, since it is fun to mix it up and experiment, I will also discuss some creative techniques.

Bearing in mind the rule that dark colors create shadows and light colors bring forward and accentuate, the correct use of contouring can transform any eye shape.

**The basic eye shapes:** round, slanted, almond, wide set, close set, and deep set.

**Various lid conditions:** puffy, dark circles and hollows, and deep tear troughs.

Eye shape is determined by a combination of the above factors. There are an infinite variety of eye descriptions. The goal of corrective eye makeup is to detract from perceived unattractive features and to enhance the best aspects of your particular eye shape.

The following explanations and illustrations for makeup application will demonstrate how to address the above concerns in order to minimize problem areas. Eyebrows are an important feature to consider as they frame the face. Correct eyebrow shape also affects the look of the eye. A good arch and a clean line open up the eye area and create a youthful look.

All eye shapes are attractive and can be enhanced with simple application techniques. Corrective eye makeup is only necessary when you feel that a certain aspect of your shape (for instance, a protruding lid, a deep-set crease, or close-set eyes) should be altered to create an illusion. I will discuss the basic applications that are suitable for most eye shapes and then address particular issues as a separate lesson.

**Eye makeup generally requires three shades:** a base color, a contour color, and a highlight color. Whatever color palette you are using, the contour color dictates the depth and intensity of the base and highlight colors. Your contour color is the guideline color. The base color is usually a nude or close to skin tone color. The highlight color complements the contour shade.

Be aware that there are "warm" and "cool" color palettes. Most people can wear both depending on the blending technique and the intensity of the application. Although skin and hair tone fall into warm and cool categories, as well, it is a myth that a warm-toned person cannot wear cool fashion and makeup colors, and vice versa.

## BASIC APPLICATION OF EYE MAKEUP

There are two basic eye makeup application styles that will suit almost every eye shape: the round and the fan. Round application is very simple. It involves applying base color over the entire lid followed by contour color in the crease—either by extending up from the lash line and into the crease, just touching the brow bone, or by shading only the crease and following the natural round shape of the crease as it meets the brow bone. In both cases, highlighter is then used to illuminate the area of the lid above the crease and into the eyebrow arch.

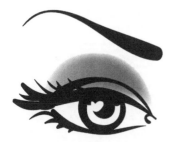 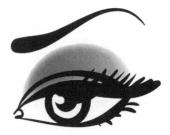

**Figure 12.1.** Round makeup application style.

Fan application takes the contour color through the crease and out towards the edge of the brow bone to the eyebrow end point. Base color and highlighter are used in the same way as in round application. The fan application starting point can also be from the base of the lashes or just in the crease line. In both types of application, the decision to take the contour color from the lash line versus just the crease depends on lid protrusion.

If you have slight to moderate lid protrusion, it is more flattering to use the contour color along the entire lid or lash line. If your lid is normal, leave the base color on the prominent part of the lid, making the eye appear to stand out. To turn any of these two basic looks into a more dramatic look, simply intensify the contour color and add a shimmer highlighter to the most prominent part of the brow bone. Apply liquid eyeliner on the upper lash line, and an additional coat of mascara to enhance the drama! In addition to these basic styles, corrective techniques and specific contouring can be added to achieve an altered aesthetic illusion.

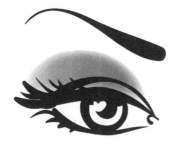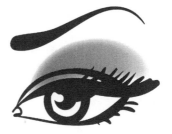

**Figure 12.2.** Fan makeup application style.

## CORRECTIVE TECHNIQUES

The following tips will help you to compensate for prominent eye shapes, including:

- Wide-set eyes
- Deep-set eyes
- Protruding lids
- Almond eyes
- Close-set eyes
- Heavy-hooded eyes
- Slanted eyes

### *WIDE-SET EYES*

Your eyes are considered wide set if the space between the inner corners of both eyes is wider than the length of one eye. It is very simple to create the illusion of narrowing the space between the eyes by contouring.

The application technique requires using a contour color along the inner bridge of the nose to create a shadow along either side of the nose from the point of the inner corner of the eye up to the inner brow point. This gives the appearance of the bridge of the nose being narrowed. To "push" the eyes further together, apply a mid-tone color from the outer point of the eye to the center point of the crease. This blurring of the outer edge gives the illusion of less distance at the outer perimeter of the eyes.

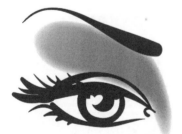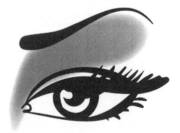

Figure 12.3. Wide-set eyes.

## CLOSE-SET EYES

If the space between your eyes is less than the length of one eye, your eyes are considered close set. Your objective will be to create the illusion of additional space between your eyes. Using a matte color that's one to two shades lighter than your lid tone, apply a contour line from the inner corner of your eye up to the inner brow point along the bridge of your nose. Begin application of the fan style from a third of the way into the crease and continue outwards to the farthest part of the lid space. The application of a shimmery highlighter at the inner corners of the eyes enhances the illusion. People with close-set eyes should also pay attention to the starting point of the inner eyebrow. Plucking the inner brows to give an extra millimeter or two of space in this area can also add to the illusion.

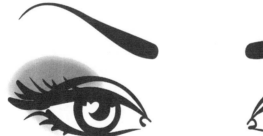

**Figure 12.4.** Close-set eyes.

## DEEP-SET EYES

Deep-set eyes have a very pronounced lid crease, which often appears as a hollow area instead of a crease line. This eye shape is also prone to under-eye circles. Deep-set eyes can be very sexy and sultry using the correct makeup application. Incorrect techniques, however, can make people with this eye shape look skeletal or tired. The most important element of the compensating technique I'm describing here is the preparation of the lid with a matte concealer to eliminate shadows in the crease.

Use a base color that is lighter than skin tone and add soft shimmer to disperse the shadow that has been created by the deep-set crease. The entire lid is then shaded with a darker contour color, starting from the lash line and extending up to the crease (without entering it). The purpose of using the darker shade is to create the illusion of recession. Combined with the effect of the highlighted crease, the lid appears more even and obvious shadows and protrusions are minimized.

The key to perfecting this seamless illusion is blending. A large eye shadow brush that is full and soft should be swept along the entire lid with a matte translucent nude eye shadow or face powder to soften the distinctive lines of the contouring shades.

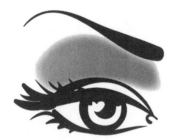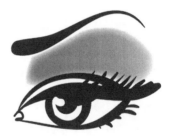

**12.5.** Deep-set eyes.

## HEAVY-HOODED EYES

Heavy-hooded eyes have a pronounced under-brow fold and an ill-defined socket crease. The best way to recognize a heavy-hooded lid is by the variance between the space above and below the crease. The upper lid is roughly two thirds of the total visible lid, whereas for most other eye shapes the ratio of the upper lid to the under-brow area above the crease is 50/50. As we age, many of us develop a heavy hood due to the weight of the fold below the eyebrow and the diminishing structural support for the brow.

Commonly known as "bedroom eyes," this eye shape can be very attractive in the right proportion, but it also has the potential to make one appear tired or prematurely aged. It can be a challenging eye shape to make up, but once you master the proper techniques it is one of the most beautiful shapes to work with. Heavy-hooded eyes are the best suited to multiple color applications and gradient blending due to the generous lid space above the crease. This is the one eye shape where I always use a minimum of three shades.

The entire lid is prepped with primer and a nude base. On the lower lid and up to the crease I apply the mid-tone color. I apply the contour color from the crease to the midway of the upper lid. Finally, a highlighter is applied from the arch of the brow and following the curve of the brow. To "open" the eye, I use either white or skin-tone eye pencils on the innermost lashes and the upper and lower lash lines, and also add color eyeliner to the outer perimeter of the lashes.

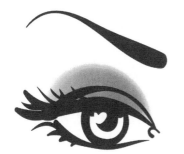 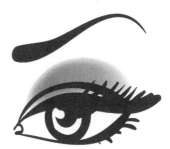

**12.6.** Heavy-hooded eyes.

## PROTRUDING LIDS

This eye shape is known for its protruding bottom eyelid. This occurs when the eyeball is prominently positioned, causing the lid to stand out. There is a simple technique that creates a dramatic illusion which can rectify the disproportionate appearance of the lid to brow bone contour. Apply a dark contour color from the upper lash line to (and ending just below) the lid crease. The lid crease is highlighted using either a matte nude or a light highlight shade coordinated with the contour color.

The width of the highlighted crease line should be wide enough to be visible when the eye is open. Above the crease and towards the brow, a medium neutral shade should be applied. In the arch of the brow, a shimmer spot of highlighter should be placed to draw an observer's eye up and away from the lower lid area. Protruding eyes always have a natural round appearance due to the shape of the eyeball.

To elongate the eye, dark liner should always be extended past the outer lash line on both the upper and lower lids. Liner must be applied in the thinnest possible line at the inner corners of the eye and sweeping outwards to its broadest point at the outer corners.

A smoky eye can be very attractive on people with this type of eye shape because of the generous lid space between upper lashes and the crease, allowing for a perfect outward sweep of liner or smoky powder shadow to be applied. The smoky eye look is great for minimizing the under-eye protrusion.

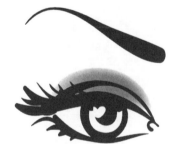 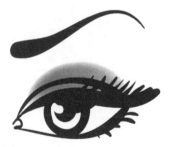

**12.7.** Protruding lids.

## *SLANTED EYES*

Slanted or "Asian" eyes typically have an almond shape that is slightly upturned at the outer corners. This eye shape often has a flat lid, meaning a very shallow crease. People with slanted eyes are a dream for every makeup artist to work with since they can wear any technique of application. Slanted eyes, by nature of the generous lid space and the lack of elevation of the lid, often have what is considered to be small eyes. In order to create the illusion of a bigger eye, one has to concentrate on the upper and lower lash lines. Apply nude, pale pink, beige, or white eyeliner to both the upper and lower inner lids to open up the eye space.

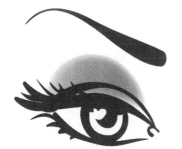 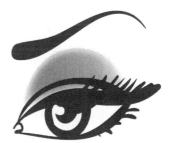

**12.8.** Slanted eyes.

## *ALMOND EYES*

Almond eyes are the standard eye shape and are therefore not usually considered a candidate for corrective techniques. Variations of the almond shape are covered in the above sections as they may have one or more of the aforementioned characteristics. They are suited to either the round or fan application of shadow.

Make adjustments according to which, if any, of the above characteristics are most prominent for you.

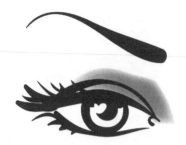 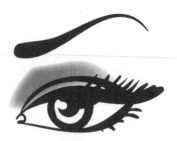

**12.9.** Almond eyes.

## LET YOUR LIPS DO THE TALKING

Bridget Bardot, Sophia Loren, Angelina Jolie, Megan Fox, Mick Jagger. Their mouths invite fantasy. Kissable lips are the most desirable feature of the face. The mouth also expresses our moods better than any other part of the face: stern lipped, tight lipped, smiling, snarling, pouting, puckering, smirking, laughing, talking, sighing, and shouting. All of our expressions are played out with our lips.

If it is true that the eyes are the windows to our souls, then the lips are the doors! Making the best of your mouth shape completes the face like no other feature. A makeup-free face can instantly be made to look glamorous with a red lipstick or soft and fresh with a nude gloss.

Full lips are considered attractive and youthful. If you are naturally thin-lipped and do not want to use fillers, lip liners are a great alternative. Using gloss to highlight the inner lip also gives the illusion of fullness.

There are four basic mouth shapes that makeup can be used to balance out: full lips, thin lips, downturned lips, and lips with no upper bow.

**Full lips:** As a makeup artist, almost all my clients wanted their lips to look fuller. Although full lips are the most desired of all lip shapes, their attractiveness is dependent on proportion and symmetry. Naturally full lips with a balanced shape look fabulous with or without lip makeup. To minimize an overly generous mouth, cover the entire lip area with foundation that perfectly matches your skin tone. In the case of the lower lip being more pronounced than the upper lip, or vice versa, draw lip liner within the lip line of the more prominent lip. On the thinner lip, apply liner to the outer edge of the lip line.

**Thin lips:** Thin lips can be easily made to look fuller. Apply the lip liner around the outer perimeter of the natural lip line to create the desired fullness. Then, apply gloss or shimmer over the lipstick shade that is being used. Place a dot of highlighter on the center area of the lips to further create the illusion of fullness. To perfectly place the highlighter, pucker your lips as if you were sucking through a straw and place the highlighter on the part of the lip that is most prominent.

**Downturned lips:** This lip shape can look sad. It is also a shape developed naturally with age, as the nasolabial folds create weight on the outer corners of the mouth. The corrective technique for this lip shape is a little tricky to master, but is very effective when done correctly. Foundation is first applied all over the lip area. Lip liner is then used along the entire lower lip line. On the upper lip line, begin your liner from the highest point of the lip at the outer corners, effectively avoiding the downturned edge of the mouth. At the outer edge of the upper lip, use a matte concealer one to two shades lighter than your foundation and blend it to blur the downturned area. Lipstick is only applied to the lip-lined area and not to the outer corners of the top lip.

**No upper bow:** Lip liner can be an easy fix for having no upper bow. Simply create the desired shape by following the natural line of the lip with lip liner and then create the illusion of a bow using the shape of the philtrum as a guide. The philtrum is the space between the nose and the mouth. The bow of the lip can be determined by measuring the depth of the groove of the philtrum.

## AGE-APPROPRIATE MAKEUP FOR WOMEN

My philosophy of age-appropriate makeup rests entirely on how old you feel! I don't like to define age by a number.

Age is an interesting phenomenon. We are certainly living in a time when the perception of age is difficult to define. Modern medicine, extended lifespans, superior nutrition, aesthetic medical procedures, and moral liberty have combined to create a healthier, more vital, and less restrictive society. We are seeing younger ages evolving to maturity faster than at any other time in history.

The proliferation of influential young celebrities, like Miley Cyrus, Lindsay Lohan, Britney Spears, Willow Smith, and Katy Perry, has created a teenage generation that dresses and behaves in a way that would have been deemed unacceptable a few decades ago. Since the days of Elvis Presley, teens have always emulated their pop idols. The difference today is the age of exposure and acceptance. As forty is the new thirty, thirteen is the new fifteen and sixteen the new eighteen.

All of these social changes are reflected through image. It is not unusual to see a woman in her fifties dating a man in his twenties, as evidenced by the emergence of the term *cougar.* It is not uncommon to visit the mall and see thirteen-year-olds with blue streaks in their hair and wearing black nails and platform shoes.

Age appropriateness has become both more and less relevant, simultaneously. It is more relevant because of the new and changing perceptions; it is less relevant because there is more freedom today than ever before.

### MAKEUP FOR YOUR TWENTIES

Your twenties represent the onset of responsibility and often a new degree of financial independence. It is the time for moving out of the parental home and establishing your own identity.

Socializing is increasingly important as new places and people become part of your experience. Even if studies continue, most twenty-somethings are getting their first jobs, either part time or as a starting point for a desired career.

Image is changing from a teen and student look to a more polished and professional one. Work and career influence our images to a great degree. Regardless of your chosen career path, makeup will always reflect your personal style. There are many women who wear uniforms, including nurses, clerks, and police-women, who express their femininity almost entirely through their makeup. It amuses and delights me when I see a woman in an austere uniform wearing false lashes, dramatic eyeliner, and red lips!

The twenties are a good time to perfect a look that works for your everyday life and can be easily adapted for social and special occasions. I personally prefer a day look that is minimal, light, soft, and fresh for the office: tinted moisturizer, neutral eye shades, and a soft color on the lips. In the same way that natural daylight shows color in its truest hue, indoor fluorescent lighting is very harsh and unflattering. For this reason, neutral and natural makeups always work best.

For an evening when you're out socially, you can increase the glam factor with shimmer and depth. Essentially, evening and special occasion makeup is always an amplified version of your signature look. Once you have identified your face, eye, and lip shapes and have learned the appropriate contouring techniques for rectifying any perceived flaws, this is the template that you should use as a basis for any occasion.

Most women develop a signature look organically by themselves as they discover their personal style. An individual woman's signature look is influenced by many factors including her beauty ideals, her upbringing, her religious observations, her profession, her creativity and self-expression. It is molded by fashion and makeup advice drawn from magazines, books, and professionals whose guidance she seeks this out.

## *MAKEUP FOR YOUR THIRTIES*

Thirty seems to scare women as much as fifty scares men! Most women see this as a defining time. If they are not in a committed relationship or have not yet had a child or achieved their professional goals, reaching this age can be a dreaded point in their lives. Many of my girlfriends and colleagues go far more graciously into their forties than turning thirty!

By the age of forty, there is a level of self-acceptance and a sense of humor that we just don't seem to have in our thirties. Also, our thirties are a time of noticing the first visible signs of aging. I assume that this is one of the main reasons why women find it hard to adjust to this decade. The thirties are actually the most wonderful of all times for a woman. According to the U.S. Centers for Disease Control and Prevention (CDC), birth rates for women in their thirties rose in 2012, while they simultaneously fell to record lows for teens and women in their twenties. The median age of marriage for women in the United States is currently twenty-seven. These statistics imply that for modern American women the thirties seem to be the decade for falling in love, getting married, and starting a family. It is also the decade when professional women have completed their studies, achieved their advanced degrees, or are settling into their chosen careers and/or starting a business. Statistically it is a unique decade because of the dynamics of marriage and starting a family. Becoming a wife and mother are still considered the most wonderful changes a woman can experience. As a childless woman in her fifth decade of life, I am not part of this demographic, but celebrate it for all those women who make up the majority of the female population. No matter what she has or has not fulfilled on her private wish list, it is a time of perfect full bloom for a woman—like a fully opened flower in its most vibrant and perfect form.

The thirties truly are a time of a woman beginning to settle into her authentic adult character. Deciding upon your studies, establishing your career, starting a business, choosing where you want to live, selecting your ideal mate, and starting a family should all be resolved in your thirties. On the proverbial road trip of life, the car should be paid for, the gas tank full, supplies and refreshments for the road picked up, and the passengers we want to travel with safely buckled in!

As far as image is concerned, this is the time when aging becomes a realization. For the first time, you will be taking note of antiaging creams and serums and spending a little more time in the mirror as you notice the appearance of fine lines. I truly believe that the thirties are when a woman's face becomes her own. It is a reflection of her spiritual, nutritional, and lifestyle choices. I find this a fascinating decade in which to study women's features.

In my experience with the beauty business, the majority of women develop their signature look in their twenties, as this is the first time they enter the workforce, begin dating more seriously, and can afford makeup and fashion. Readers of fashion magazines like *Elle, Cosmopolitan, Allure,* and *InStyle* are predominantly women aged 25–35. The twenties are when a young woman is establishing her adult signature style, which evolves from that point onwards. Your signature makeup look does not need to be altered in your thirties since your face shape won't change dramatically. Depending on hormonal changes, skin condition, certain medications, and emotional or anxiety-related issues, you may consider changing your foundation. The eye area may require a little more concealer, as well.

## MAKEUP FOR YOUR FORTIES

The big Four-Oh! If forty is the new thirty, we may not need to address this decade at all! Women are increasingly taking better care of their skin—and it is truly evident. This particular age group is becoming harder to distinguish. Consider all of the supermodels of the 1980s, including Cindy Crawford (48), Naomi Campbell (44), Christy Turlington (45), Claudia Schiffer (43), Linda Evangelista (49), and Elle MacPherson (51). Also the female cast of the television hit, Friends: Jennifer Aniston (45), Courtney Cox (50), and Lisa Kudrow (50), and movie stars like Cameron Diaz (42), Julia Roberts (47), Pamela Anderson (47), Salma Hayek (48), Gwyneth Paltrow (42), Catherine Zeta-Jones (45), Elizabeth Hurley (49), Jennifer Lopez (45), Monica Bellucci (50), Halle Berry (48), Sarah Jessica Parker (49), and Nicole Kidman (47). It is stunning to see how these women look today, now that they are in their mid to late forties, or in a few cases, their early fifties.

Although the aforementioned women were undeniably magnificent in their twenties and thirties, there is something almost sexier about them due to how they have aged. The experience and confidence of a forty-something-year-old woman who still looks as good as she did in her twenties or thirties is appealing. Whether or not these women have had various procedures, their beauty lies in the natural appearance of their maintenance. Your image and makeup from your thirties to your forties—and even up to your fifties—shouldn't change dramatically if you are taking care of your skin and living a healthy lifestyle.

## MAKEUP FOR YOUR FIFTIES

The fifties are when we notice the most obvious changes in our facial features and bodies. In spite of lifestyle choices and what is available to us with surgical and aesthetic advancements, the aging process is inevitable. Due to hormonal changes and the natural slowing of cell renewal, many functions previously taken for granted become issues that we begin to notice. Disease and chronic illness top our awareness as we, as well as others in our age bracket, more previously will experience ill health or reduced functions. Our recovery time increases after physical exertion or a bout of the flu, and this can be a reminder to us, especially if we have let ourselves go fitness-wise, that our bodies are no longer operating at peak performance. Energy levels can diminish and sleep problems can develop, too.

Of course, there is the Madonna phenomenon. Madonna (56) has single-handedly redefined the meaning of age management and how to be vital and energetic, healthy, relevant, sexy, and a powerhouse at any age. Whether or not you agree with her on-stage antics or find her athletic frame attractive, she undeniably has the energy and vitality of a person twenty years younger because of the effort she's put into her fitness. Her image is edgy and modern, and her facial features, while certainly having had the benefit of procedures, appear to be naturally youthful. Other superb examples of beautiful celebrities retaining their youthful appearance in their fifties are: Heather Locklear (53), Michelle Pfeiffer (55), Meg Ryan (53), Christie Brinkley (60), Demi Moore (52), Kim Basinger (60), Sharon Stone (56), Annette Benning (56), Ellen DeGeneres (56), Tilda Swinton (54), Emma Thompson (55), and Kim Cattrall (58).

We are living in an age of ageless transformation. For all of the celebrities and supermodels that I have mentioned, there is a whole generation of women who are looking as good as they did when they were ten or fifteen years younger.

As a result of age management and our healthier lifestyle, we are enjoying a greater quality of life than ever before. There is a whole new generation of actively dating older singles, for instance, as evidenced by the proliferation of online dating websites catering to people over forty. The divorce rate in Western culture has made it more important than ever for people in this age bracket to have an image that others will find attractive. Women should be aware that, at this age, you do not want to appear as though you are trying to look younger. It is far more attractive to be confident and happy with your appearance.

As a makeup artist, I am exposed to the psychology of women at various stages of life and experience. When a woman is sitting with you in an intimate environment, with her face natural and unmade up, an honesty and vulnerability emerges. In discussing openly what she considers her best and worst features, the conversation reveals her confidence, self-knowledge, wisdom, and her insecurities. I am always amazed at how self-critical most women can be. They draw attention to perceived flaws that would be almost nonexistent to a casual observer.

I find that our emotional state directly affects our self-confidence. The most gorgeous woman, for instance, would likely feel unattractive if she discovered her husband was cheating on her. Women who have gained weight feel a lack of sex appeal and often will try to compensate for it by either dressing a certain way or changing their hair or makeup style. Some react to weight gain by losing interest in their grooming altogether. Also, a lack of understanding of menopausal symptoms can lead to depression and frustration.

Due to mood swings, sleep disturbances, and memory issues they experienced (which are by no means universally experienced by women in menopause), some of my clients have felt like they were going crazy. I ask them to imagine that they have a protracted case of premenstrual tension and this makes them giggle! We talk, share, and laugh as I make them up and, miraculously, they leave the chair feeling happy, confident, and hopeful. Why? Makeup is transformative. Can you imagine if your favorite celebrities made appearances without styled hair and makeup? The fantasy and illusion would be destroyed! At this age it is important for women to make the best of themselves in order to feel good.

Interestingly, I have found that this decade of makeup warrants a return to a much younger look—wearing makeup and hair almost the way you did in your late teens and twenties: soft natural peaches and corals, neutrals, and nudes on eyes and lips. Hair looks gorgeous shoulder length and tousled. My image inspirations for this age are Michelle Pfeiffer and Elle MacPherson. Madonna, when not performing, is often photographed makeup free in her workout gear. This is when I think she looks most youthful. Annette Benning and Meg Ryan's untidy cropped hairstyles give them the appearance of casual rebellion. It's a young illusion that is very attractive.

Other people's opinions do matter. This is why we love a compliment and find a negative comment hurtful. The happy medium is to find your own place of comfort with your look and to be aware of the reactions that you invite. If you get it right, there should be an overwhelming positive response.

It always fascinates me when people, particularly celebrities, say, "I don't care what other people think of me," and then do everything they can to draw attention to themselves. The truth is that we do dress to impress. We do care about our images and are sensitive to the responses we get. As we age, it becomes both less and more important to us: less because of our confidence, self-knowledge, wisdom, and acceptance of our bodies; and more because new insecurities surface as the aging process begins to show. Striving to create a healthy balance is the best advice we can give.

## MAKEUP FOR YOUR SIXTIES

The sixties have never been sexier! Meryl Streep (65), Sigourney Weaver (65), Helen Mirren (68), Susan Sarandon (67), Glenn Close (67), Diane Keaton (67), Jessica Lange (65), Anjelica Huston (63), Lauren Hutton (70), Goldie Hawn (68), and Cher (68) show us what a beautiful and sexy decade this can be! It is wonderful to see so many examples of women in their sixties looking beautiful and retaining their elegance and grace. This is a time when younger generations are looking for you to share your advice and guidance based on your years of life experience. I love my clients in this age group—they are so interesting and informative. From the perfect cookie recipe to running a multinational organization, their lifetime of trial and error makes for a fascinating encounter. As the generation that saw the birth of the women's liberation movement, it is a perfect age to fully appreciate and take advantage of this historic time of women's social development.

Your image in your sixth decade should appear to be effortless. Whether for your everyday look or for a special occasion, you know what works best for you. There is a great freedom in accepting where you are in your life and allowing your image to fit seamlessly with your personality. I enjoy when my clients of this age group surprise me with a bold new hair color or by changing their eyeglasses to a funky shape or color.

An interesting statistic has emerged within this age group for both men and women relating to sexual activity. The introduction of Viagra and other medications to treat erectile dysfunction, coupled with the divorce rate and the improved health and fitness of this demographic, have resulted in the phenomenon that people in their sixties are more sexually active now than at any other time in history. In keeping with this trend, women are not only looking to maintain their image, but to develop their sex appeal. Many of my clients in this age group have told me that they are dating again for the first time in years. Some sadly lost their loved ones. Others divorced for different reasons.

How we look truly affects how we feel. It also influences how people respond to us. With each changing decade we should have a look that works for that particular phase of our lives.

*MAKEUP FOR THE YEARS BEYOND . . .*

A seventy-three-year old client once told me that the only thing you need to work on in your seventies is your sense of humor. I remember her well because we laughed pretty much throughout our entire makeup session. This woman had a twinkle in her eye. Of the countless interesting and beautiful women that I have had the pleasure of making over, she made a lasting impression on me. She helped me find clarity to a conundrum that I had been wrestling with in the beauty business for some time. Dealing with women every day and seeing how their image constantly alternates between making them happier and more confident to being more insecure and depressed, I have often wondered if I was helping to improve this condition or part of the very machinery that was creating the insecurities that it claimed to remedy. This particular woman helped me realize that remaining faithful to a routine that you do throughout your life, such as wearing makeup, is an overwhelmingly positive act.

Women are fortunate to have a ritual available to them that can transform their appearance and make them feel more beautiful. No matter what age or phase of your life you are enjoying, everything is brighter with a little color.

## YOUR SIGNATURE LOOK: SPECIAL OCCASIONS

A first date, a prom, a job interview, being a bride or a bridesmaid, receiving an award, presenting your doctoral dissertation, an anniversary dinner, or a christening, a lifetime achievement honor, appearing on television to discuss your latest book—we all want to look our very best for memorable events such as these! We also want to make sure that if we are going to be photographed, the image is going to be one that we are happy to share and want to look at for years to come with pride and fond memories. I have to say, though, that those pictures that we all have from when we really got it wrong have priceless value when we need a laugh!

Special occasions are an opportunity to treat yourself to the services of a professional. Going to a hairstylist and a makeup artist can make you feel like a star preparing for the red carpet! It is not necessary to pay for the services of a makeup artist when all department and specialty makeup stores have trained makeup artists who will happily provide their services for free with no obligation to purchase products.

Without exception, I use false eyelashes for special occasion makeup. No matter how thick or long your own lashes are, the perfection of shape provided by a false lash set is unparalleled. It doubles your volume and increases length.

If you are doing your makeup yourself, always stick to your signature look and add elements that amplify the look or co-ordinate with your outfit. A little touch, such as matching the shade of eyeliner to the predominant color of your outfit, some-times creates a more polished look.

The look also varies according to the occasion. Makeup for a job interview will look nothing like the look you would wear to a prom. Likewise, bridal makeup is different from bride to brides-maid and for the mother of the bride.

My all-time favorite bridal look is soft and romantic with smoky eyes. Makeup for bridesmaids is dependent on the color of the dress. Occasion makeup is your signature look with add-ed glamour or drama.

For a professional interview, you want a polished, profession-al look—no shimmers or gloss. A nude eye shadow with minimal mascara and a bold red lip, however, can make a powerful state-ment and create a lasting impression.

Photography requires variable consideration. Certainly, matte foundation is key. Shimmers can show up as greasy shine when lights are flashing.

Whenever you are doing a variation of your signature look, it all begins with your basic application style—round or fan. Then, simply use different shades, darker eyeliner, and false eyelashes, adding shimmer or gloss to suit the occasion and outfit.

## FASHIONS AND THE SEASONS

Seasons affect our moods and require us to change our image by dressing appropriately for the changing weather. Certainly in the world of media, the announcement of a new season has more to do with fashion than temperature! Each season heralds new "must-haves" and "don't dos." This color is in; that one is out. Brown is the new black—no, navy is the new black. No, grey is the new black! Pastels are the new white—no, nudes are the new white and blush is the new beige! It can be very confusing.

Just as we get one trend right, the fashion world announces its death and the birth of a new one that we need to catch up with! Along with every new seasonal fashion collection, there are "bridge collections" just to keep it interesting and confuse us a little more.

In tandem with the fashion designers, makeup companies launch a look for every season. With each fashion and cosmetic house creating its own interpretation of the "look of the season," it is virtually impossible to cover it all. I like to keep up with the key trends for a season—the general color mood and the global inspiration behind the trend—rather than get into all of the interpretations.

Have fun with what inspires you in a particular season. You may be in the mood for a nautically inspired summer, wearing sailor stripes and cropped white jeans, and sporting red lipstick. Or, you may love the pastel and sorbet colors and want pretty pink eyes and candy-floss colored lips. Summer vacation may see you bronzed and wanting to wear coral eye shadow and turquoise eyeliner.

Winter could make you yearn for soft, smoky brown eye shadow and warm cranberry colored lips. Fashion and makeup are very mood driven, so I always guide my clients to experiment with the trends. It is also wise to buy cheaper mass-market brands of makeup that are usually right on trend for what are going to be the big sellers.

## WHAT YOU SEE IS WHAT YOU GET

After mastering your signature look, and considering all the influences throughout the decades that have affected how you present yourself to the world—such as the changing seasons and the passing trends—the one constant is that you are still YOU.

You may have looked differently at certain times, experimented with new trends and experienced life-changing events, but those are external considerations. Your soul, character, and personality do not change—they evolve. The many women who have sat in my makeup chair have taught me that as we age, the one real benefit is that we better understand ourselves, life, and the world, and can settle into being who we really are.

The highest plateau we can reach in life is to be truly happy. No matter your financial, professional, or other achievements, what do they mean if you are not happy? I love how being associated with the beauty industry has exposed me to many truly wise women. I sincerely hope you find your true beauty in life—the beauty of acceptance, peace, and contentment—and that you look and feel gorgeous doing it.

# CHAPTER 13

# Be Youthful

---

W hen patients come to our clinic for a cosmetic consultation, I never bother to ask their chronological ages. It's of little importance to me. What is important to me is how young (or old) they act and feel. Only then do I look at their faces to see if they have acquired any elderly looking features, including signs of facial descent or volume loss.

Age is not a number to me, but rather a state of mind. I have seen some eighty-something-year-old women that have more youth and vitality than women in their fifties. I have also seen more wrinkles on some thirty-something-year-old women than on some of my sixty-something-year-old patients. I am convinced that people really do think themselves into old age. If you believe that once you reach a certain age or milestone you're going to start aging, then you absolutely will. The subconscious mind is such a powerful force that it has the ability to create and shape our experience of reality. You can literally will every cell in your body to start to age and perish—or you can will the opposite. It's your choice.

The truth is that we are living longer. This is a fact! However, what we should really be trying to do is to add more life to our years—not just more years to our lives. I am amazed when my eighty-year-old patients tell me that they get up every day at six in the morning to play tennis, golf, or swim. One seventy-five year-old patient does CrossFit every day with his seventy-year-old wife. These people are not only physically strong, they also look years younger than their chronological ages. I used to think that your eighties were about waiting for your turn to hear the fat lady sing! This mentality is the reason why certain people, once they reach a certain age, stop trying to stay young. They just re-tire from life because they believe it's their time to decline.

While working as a hospice physician, I became interested in learning about end of life care and human behavior around death. During my research, I came across a book written in 1958 by Arnold A. Hutschnecker, M.D., *The Will to Live*. The premise of this book is that the mind and the body are interconnected: "We age, not by years, but rather by events and our emotional reactions to them." I agree.

For example, I have witnessed that some of my patients age rapidly within a few months of going through a divorce. How-ever, I have also seen other patients who look younger after a divorce. Our perception of our situation is what causes us to age or blossom. The old adage "You can't teach an old dog new tricks" is absolutely false! It should say, "You cannot teach an old dog new tricks—if the dog thinks it's old."

During medical school, I had a few classmates in their late fifties and early sixties who had decided to go back to school to become doctors. Their learning capacities were as good as any of us youngsters in the class—and maybe better. They had the wisdom and the discipline that sometimes come only with age. If my eighty-something-year-old patients can get up ev-ery morning to play tennis, then there is no real physiological evidence that we should give up on our personal goals and in-terests once we reach a certain age, either. A person grows old when he or she allows the body to become sedentary. Like I tell all of my patients, "If you don't give your body a reason to re-generate, then your body can only degenerate."

A close friend of mine called one day to tell me that he had TiVo-ed an episode of Oprah that was going to blow my mind. I thought, *Great, Oprah is giving away more cars!* To my surprise, however, she was interviewing the one and only Raquel Welch. I had already heard through the grapevine that she still looked fantastic, but when Welch walked on the set, I was stunned! She looked better at almost seventy than when she had done her last interview with Oprah in the 1980s. She did not just look good for her age—she looked incredible for any age!

When speaking about her secrets for staying youthful physi-cally, mentally, and emotionally, instead of talking about lotions, potions, or plastic surgery, she emphasized that the best way to stay youthful is never to retire from the game of life. The in-terview reminded me of the response given by almost every-one who looks fantastic in their later decades in response to my question of how they look so youthful. They all tell me, "I never think of myself as being 'old.'"

Oprah quoted from a page of Welch's book, *Raquel: Beyond the Cleavage.* It states that the word *old* is the "only dirty word left in the English language." Nothing could be closer to the truth. In our youth- and image-conscious society, calling some-one old is a terrible insult. Sometimes I worry whenever people think that my chronological age is more than twenty-something, even though twenty-something is half of my actual chronologi-cal age. It is absolutely ridiculous!

However, I use these moments as an opportunity to spread the word to my patients that age is more a state of mind than an actual number. We should all feel blessed to have the opportuni-ty to have another birthday each year. I, for one, intend never to consider myself old, no matter how many birthdays I've had or how old I may appear to others. The motto in my clinic is: "The older we get, the younger we look." We cannot possibly be the age that our birth certificate, driver's license, or passport says we are because we look, act, and feel years younger.

Today, when we think about ageless beauties, we think about Suzanne Somers, Joan Collins, and Raquel Welch—iconic figures that inspire us to look great at any age! Their male counterparts are celebrities like Pierce Brosnan, Sting, and Denzel Washington. As public figures and sex symbols, when they were in their prime they had a need to maintain their youthful appearances. Similarly, many actors, actresses, and models manage to look younger than their actual chronological ages. In Hollywood, where you are judged even more harshly when your looks start to fade, there is a real need to maintain your youth and vitality at all costs. For the rest of us, without a professional imperative to stay youthful as the years pass, aging may come a lot faster than we would like it to, especially if we believe it will. We either surrender to cultural expectations, give up making a consistent effort to stay vital, and let our capacities lapse—essentially giving up on life—or we never learn to do the right things to age well and gracefully in the first place.

We are conditioned to believe that old age starts after we reach a certain age, whether that is when we reach fifty or sixty, or after retirement. If you are a woman, old age supposedly comes right after menopause. Yet one of my most amazing looking patients told me that for her life started at age 60. Constance is a very lively woman, and at age sixty-five she has a better face and body than many forty-year-old women who come to my practice. I told her that I was writing a book and wanted to share her secrets with my readers on how to stay so young looking.

Constance believes in prevention. Her secrets to staying youthful are working on having a good posture, using bioidentical hormones, and tackling any little changes that she sees in her face and body. She is a testament that aging well is directly related to how old you are when you start to take care of yourself. If you understand the aging face, then you don't allow it to drop and shift. If you want a young and healthy body, you can only achieve it with a healthy diet, regular physical exercise, and by incorporating yoga or Pilates to literally keep up your youthful posture.

Not long ago, I took a trip to Peru to see the Incan ruins of Machu Picchu. Everyone I know who has gone raves about the spiritual energy that is tangible there. Before going to the ruins, we had to stay for one day in the city of Cusco to acclimate to the high altitude. While walking through the streets of the city, I saw many indigenous women with sun-weathered skin. Their deep facial wrinkles and saggy skin made them look very old, but their bodies were as strong as bulls. These indigenous women walk for miles and miles under the fierce sun with their alpacas carrying their goods and crafts to sell in the city.

Although they have no need or concern for the beauty or youthfulness of their faces, they do need to have the physical strength and endurance to walk for miles under the hot South American sun. They walk with good posture and pace, and their physical strength is as strong as any youngster in their clans. Observing these strong, elderly women—some well into their eighties—helped me to understand that if we continue to use our bodies and have a reason to stay fit, our bodies will remain strong and limber no matter what our age.

The mistake that most of us make, which tends to accelerate the aging process, is to believe that once we reach our retirement it is acceptable to have a sedentary life. It should be quite the opposite: The period after retirement is when we should take advantage of the extra time at our disposal to work on our minds, bodies, and spirits. Most people use their retirement years to go on cruises and other vacations. That's quite all right, but it's not going to help the body to stay young. The only way to maintain a good posture and strong muscles is by habitually stretching and exercising.

Retirement should not equate to getting to eat whatever we want. When I lived in Delray Beach, Florida, I would see signs in many restaurants for early bird specials, catering to all of the senior citizens that have come to Florida to live a life of leisure. The food is more affordable during these specials, but it is also very rich—or should I say, unhealthy. It's a big social event for the seniors of the nearby communities. I sometimes would glance at their plates and gasp when I saw the types of foods that they were eating. Later life is when we should be watching our diets! Instead, the diets of these seniors were actually accelerating the aging process and promoting all kind of diseases.

The will to stay youthful has promoted great advances in medicine, cosmetics, and nutrition. In this book, we've managed to review most of the technological, cosmeceutical, and medical advancements available to us today; however, with the exception of our discussion of antioxidants in fruits and vegetables until this chapter, we have only touched lightly upon the ways nutrition can help us to add more youth, health, and vitality to our years.

During my research about diet and nutrition, I came across countless diets and hordes of nutritional advice. Every expert seems to have his or her own opinion about which diet has the most benefit for the human body. It was as confusing as trying to choose an eye cream in a department store.

Not long before giving up on the subject, I ran into a patient while on my way to my Pilates class. She gave me small packages of a powder product containing green superfoods like spirulina, kelp, wheatgrass, adaptogenic herbs, and spinach and other leafy green vegetables, among other ingredients. After doing some of my own research into this type of green drink (there are many good brands), I became convinced that I had found a path to nutritional enlightenment. The premise of the diet I now adhere to is that eating foods that restore and maintain the acid-alkaline pH balance in the blood and tissue help establish the perfect internal environment for a healthy body.

Every living cell in the human body is surrounded by a vital force that allows for cell-to-cell communication, energy production, and homeostasis. This invisible, but tangible force is the human electromagnetic field. It behaves like a fluid and is the source of all life. This field changes shape and strength in conjunction with physiological and psychological changes. For this reason, it can be easily affected by changes or disturbances in temperature, pH levels, and emotions.

The human body has an intricate biochemistry that allows us to generate an electromagnetic field that is vital for the regulation of our inner environment. This electromagnetic field, in conjunction with the brain, heart, liver, and kidneys, is responsible for keeping every cell in our body alive and healthy. In order to maintain this electromagnetic field, our bodies must have a certain acid-alkaline pH balance. Using a scale of 1 to 14, with 1 being extremely acidic and 14 being extremely basic, or alkaline, the human body functions best at a pH level of about 7.36 (slightly basic). A small shift of only one or two points on this scale can be detrimental to our health and limit our survival.

The maintenance of the body's pH is as important as the maintenance of the core temperature of the body. With any drastic change in pH level or temperature in the body, death is sure to follow.

Fortunately, the human body is designed to compensate for any slight change in temperature or pH level. However, as we have evolved and our diets and lifestyles have changed, we have become less and less capable of maintaining the perfect pH level at the micromolecular level in the tissue. Due to both the demands of our industrialized, high-tech lives and the mass-produced, processed food products that we so frequently intake, we are living very acidic lifestyles.

It is no secret that our emotions are the number one source of acid production in the body. We've all experienced the discomfort of being stressed or upset. I remember hearing my grandmother saying to my cousins and me, when we were misbehaving, "You guys make me feel so acidic—you are going to put me in the grave before my time!" Not until learning about the acid-alkaline diet did her words make any sense to me. Acidity leads to inflammation, which leads to physical responses that can be healing in the short term, but in the long term are destructive to tissues of the body.

By avoiding unnecessary stress and developing better coping mechanisms and learning strategies to interrupt the stress response and promote relaxation, such as meditation, exercise, communing with nature, or even by taking a few deep breaths when we feel emotionally triggered, we can maintain a healthy acid-alkaline biochemistry in our bodies.

All the technological advances of recent years were supposed to free us from having too much stress. We have better transportation, computers, fax machines, smartphones, televisions, and more information than we could want at the tips of our fingers. However, because we are excessively connected to our technological devices we're spending less and less time enjoying the outdoors or being with our friends and families. I see many people having dinner together in restaurants who are texting and checking their emails rather than interacting. It's ludicrous! Some recent research studies have claimed that extended sitting, as we do to watch television, drive a car, or use a personal computer, is more hazardous to our health than smoking cigarettes. As a result of the demands and deficits of the modern lifestyle, stress is putting many of us into our graves far too early.

Our diets are the second leading cause of acid formation and accumulation in our tissues. The human body was designed to assimilate nutrients drawn right from Mother Nature: fruits and vegetables, which are alkaline. Today, most of our foods are mass-produced and loaded with preservatives, hormones, pesticides, and other chemicals. Those chemicals aren't nutritious—they're toxic to the body—and they can even interfere with the absorption of vitamins, minerals, and phytonutrients.

In addition, we make very poor food choices. We have a tendency to go for meats, starches, and sweets, which are acidic. The poor veggies sit sadly on the side of our plates, as if they were put there merely for decoration. We overindulge in acid-forming foods and do little to increase our alkaline reserves or to cleanse our bodies from acid-forming residues. As our bodies gradually become overloaded with acid residues, our health begins to deteriorate.

Most people are convinced that germs (bacteria and viruses) are the main cause of the diseases that tend to afflict the human population. Nevertheless, it is a fact that although germs may play an important role in several disease processes, disease can only occur in a body that is weakened by acid-forming residues or has genetic deficiencies.

During the flu season, some people choose to get the flu vaccine while many do not. Nevertheless, not everyone gets the flu, whether or not they received the vaccination. Do we actually believe that the flu virus waits every year for the holidays to come and invade us? The flu viruses do not pack their bags and migrate every season to ruin the holidays for us. They are always around us, but individuals who have weakened immune systems (from an accumulation of acid-forming residues) are the ones most likely to manifest an illness.

There are a lot of factors that contribute to the accumulation of acids in the body during the holidays. First of all, we tend to be stressed and worried about money. In addition, during the holidays our bodies are also busy trying to cope with and endure cold temperatures. Finally, we have perhaps the worst diets of the year during the holidays. Our consumption of alcoholic beverages and overindulgence in acid-producing foods and beverages cause the internal environment of the body to become compromised, leading to a weakened immune system. Therefore, rather than being attacked by the flu virus, it is more that we make ourselves into perfect hosts for the legendary flu virus to make its home in our bodies.

In a renowned 1950 journal article, "Global Strategy in Preventative Medicine," F.K. Meyer, M.D., writes, "Human history shows that the root of epidemics is not the disease but poor health."

A body that accumulates a lot of acid residue in the blood and tissues is polluted and therefore capable of attracting and hosting all kinds of disease-causing germs. The cholera epidemic of the 1800s that Dr. Meyer was discussing is a great illustration of how polluting our environment can lead to diseases that can potentially spin out of control and affect millions of people in a relatively short period of time.

Cholera-causing bacteria were able to spread rapidly throughout Europe and later in America due to the inadvertent transport of polluted bilge water, mainly from British ships. Of those who contracted the disease, most of those with poor health didn't survive. This teaches us how it is vitally important to keep our external and internal environments free of pollution so that we can enjoy harmonious and healthy lives.

The first time I heard about acid-alkaline balance was almost fifteen years ago during medical school when an older gentleman who had come in for his yearly physical told me that he was supposed to be dead. He had been diagnosed with throat cancer that was so advanced that doctors advised him and his wife to seek palliative care at a hospice facility. He had learned about alkalizing the body in his research about cancer and alternative medicine, and having nothing to lose, he put himself in an alternative medical center where he could detoxify and alkalize his body. He became disease free—and continued to be so for over twenty years. Later, he was instructed to drink coral calcium for the rest of his natural life to keep his alkaline reserves at their maximum levels. The more research I did on this subject, the more testimonials I discovered about the power of alkalizing the body to help fight cancer and other illnesses.

I was still skeptical, however, until I saw how a close friend with breast cancer had benefited from alkalizing her body. She went to a well-known naturopathic doctor in South Africa. After alkalizing her body, her tumors shrank significantly to the amazement of her oncologists. The premise of the treatment she received was that cancerous cells can neither grow nor survive in an alkalized environment. Witnessing my friend's ordeal and the happy outcome helped me to appreciate the importance of a diet that increases the alkaline reserves in the body and neutralizes the acid residues in our tissues.

The human body is like an intricate power plant that generates an enormous amount of energy via electrical reactions. These reactions keep every cell, tissue, and organ alive and functioning. As with any other power plant, waste is produced from the generation of this energy. This waste contributes to the formation of an acid ash that accumulates in the tissues. If too much acid waste accumulates in the tissues without neutralization, it can lead to sickness.

Remember, every cell in the body needs an environmental pH level that is close to 7.36. If there is a constant accumulation of acid residue, the cells will do everything in their power to survive. This can lead to cell mutations or even malignancy.

Cancerous cells are native cells in a particular organ or tissue that mutate, become aggressive, and then get out of control. The body has different mechanisms that can be used in order to maintain the proper pH level in the tissues. One of these mechanisms is to use the alkaline reserves in the body to neutralize the acids. However, if we are constantly creating more acids than can be neutralized, the alkaline reserves will be consumed and it will be even more difficult to neutralize the additional acids.

It takes four parts of alkalinity to neutralize one part of acid. Once alkaline reserves are used up, another backup mechanism is used to store the extra acids in the body fat.

We all have our own inherited genetic weaknesses. Some people are prone to strokes and heart attacks. Other people may have a family history of Alzheimer's disease or hypertension. It is a known fact that acid accumulation will do the most damage in the areas of our inherited weaknesses. Therefore, people who have a predisposition to a particular type of genetic disease should do the best they can via diet and exercise to keep the body's pH level at its optimum in every tissue.

It's our obligation to do everything in our power to decrease the amount of acid in our tissues. Finding a way to cope with stress and exercising regularly are a good start. In addition, being conscientious of the types of foods that we eat is very important for maintaining the proper acid-alkaline balance in our bodies. I've made some changes in my own diet since becoming enlightened on this subject. I do my best to eat 80 percent of my meals from alkaline-forming foods and 20 percent from acid-forming foods. I also purposefully detox my body from time to time so that I can get rid of acid-forming wastes. There are plenty of natural ways to detox the body. These include juicing with raw fruits and vegetables, doing hot yoga, and having colonics. Many gastroenterologists and family physicians agree that colon hydrotherapy is a great method to keep the body in good health.

Since I began to detox regularly, I have noticed a positive impact on my overall state of well-being. Normal aging occurs when the cells in our body lose their capability to regenerate. It is imperative that we create an ideal biochemical environment in our bodies to promote healthy cell growth and regeneration.

As a dermatologist, I can only give a brief explanation and some advice about how to obtain a pH-balanced diet. Two books that have really helped me to understand this concept in great depth are *Alkalize or Die* by Theodore A. Baroody, D.C, N.D., Ph.D., and *The Acid-Alkaline Diet for Optimum Health* by Christopher Vasey, N.D. These books contain a wealth of knowledge that can help you to choose the right foods to achieve and maintain the appropriate pH level in your tissues for optimum health.

Our ability to stay youthful is also influenced by the type of people with whom we surround ourselves. Surrounding yourself with peers who mainly discuss disease, medical appointments, getting old, and death will only speed up your aging process. If you have these kinds of friends, I'm not saying that you cannot love them or spend quality time with them. Just don't join the

"Alta Caca High-mileage Club." Whomever you spend the most time with is who you become, so select a peer group that thinks and speaks positively and for whom staying healthy and looking youthful are significant values.

It is important to avoid synchronizing your internal clock with peers that have retired from life or who have a pessimistic view about the golden years. I often use the phenomenon of synchronous menstruation in women to explain the impact of picking our peer groups. Just as women who have been living together start to have coinciding periods, people who spend a lot of time together start to think, speak, and believe similarly.

It is also important to surround yourself with younger or young-acting peers. They will inspire you to try to keep healthy and fit, and it can even cause your internal clock to slow down a bit.

Whether we like it or not, the opinions of others affect the ways in which we perceive ourselves and how we live our lives. It is said that "birds of a feather flock together," so it is important that we choose peers who are optimistic and have a zest for life. Researchers and doctors agree that people with a positive outlook and young spirits are less susceptible to the usual physical ills of middle age.

I chose *Be Youthful* as the title of this book because this phrase resonates with the messages that I am trying to convey. In order to be youthful, we should first start with the soul. Yes, you have been presented with a lot of important and useful information about lasers, fillers, Botox, cosmeceuticals, and makeup in this book. Even so, staying youthful takes a lot more than that. A soul that's full of resentment, depression, anxiety, anger, or fear is a soul whose body will experience accelerated aging.

Cultivating faith, hope, gratitude, joy, excitement, and appreciation, on the other hand, decelerates the aging process. The combination of these characteristics generates a life force in us that keeps us young and vital. They create a state of mind that adds enthusiasm, health, and happiness to our years. Those who manage to harness their life force age more slowly and live with more vitality than others.

# Acknowledgments

My career is dedicated to being of service. Now I feel fortunate to be given the opportunity to acknowledge those who have taught me, worked beside me, assisted me, collaborated with me, and befriended me to enable me to fulfill my purpose. This book represents the culmination of a lifetime of learning and the cooperative skills, focused efforts, and shared vision of many talented individuals. While it is impossible to mention by name each person who has contributed to *Be Youthful*, I take this opportunity to express my gratitude and heartfelt thanks to the following:

My mentors in my dermatology residency program at Nova Southeastern University: Robert Berg, M.D., Les Rosen, M.D., Brad Glick, D.O., Richard Rubenstein, M.D., Marty Zaiac, M.D., and Franciso Kerdel, M.D.

My colleagues Theresa Cao, D.O., and Jerry Obed, D.O., who kindly reviewed the contents of this book. Of course, any remaining errors are mine, not theirs.

My dear friend Loren Psaltis, for her generous contribution of her expert insights on makeup for the chapter "Color Me

Perfect," as well as the illustrations that accompany her advice. Without Loren's encouragement and example as an author, I probably would not have taken on this project in the first place. Special thanks to the team at Lincoln Square Books LLC: my publishing consultant, copyeditor, and project manager, Stephanie Gunning; her partner Peter Rubie; researcher Claire Putsche; indexer Andrea Jones; and cover and interior designer Gus Yoo. You made my publishing experience easy and fun. Paul Lipton, I truly appreciate your introduction to Stephanie and LSB.

Editors Alex Obed and Alejandro Suarez, I am indebted to you for helping me organize my thoughts and polish my words in early drafts of my manuscript. Jake Campbell, thank you for helping me with research.

Thanks to the following individuals for their assistance in creating the perfect cover: Photographer Antonio Cuellar, for the image on the cover. Photo shoot producer Camilo Morales. Rich Goren, for your input on the cover art.

I am grateful to my patients. Ultimately, you are my motivation. On a daily basis, you inspire me to continue looking for new and better ways to reverse the signs of aging.

# Resources

Shino Bay Cosmetic Dermatology, Plastic Surgery,
and Laser Institute
350 Las Olas Boulevard, Suites 110 and 120
Fort Lauderdale, FL. 33301
(954) 765-3005
http://shinobayderm.com

## CONNECT VIA THE SOCIAL NETWORKS

Twitter.com/Shino_Bay
Facebook.com/ShinoBayDerm
LinkedIn.com/pub/shino-bay-aguilera/86/872/157
Instagram.com/ShinoBay

## PRODUCTS

### *HUMAN GROWTH FACTORS*

TNS Recovery Complex (www.skinmedica.com); through doctors' offices only

Neocutis PSP Bio Cream, Bio Serum, and Journée (www.neocutis.com)

### *ANIMAL-DERIVED GROWTH FACTORS*

Tensage Intensive Serum ampoules and moisturizing creams (www.biopelle.com); through doctors' offices only

### *PLANT-DERIVED GROWTH FACTORS*

Obagi Gentle Rejuvenation systems (www.obagi.com); through doctors' offices only

Kinerase skincare products (www.ulta.com)

PyratineXR Skin Cream systems (www.pyratine.com)

Pyratine-6 Soft Skin Cream (www.walgreens.com)

### *OXYGEN-BASED TREATMENTS*

Dermacyte Oxygen Concentrate products (www.dermacyteUS.com); through doctors' offices only

### *OXYGEN-BASED COSMETICS*

Oxygenetix Post Procedure Foundation; through doctors' offices only

### *ANTI-GLYCATION TECHNOLOGY*

A.G.E. Interrupter (www.SkinCeuticals.com); through doctors' offices only

Supplamine (Dynamis Skin Science; 1-877-682-7949)

## POWDER-BASED SUNSCREEN

Colorescience Sunforgettable SPF 50 Sunscreen
(www.sephora.com)

## LOTION-BASED SUNSCREEN

Shino Bay Cosmetic Solutions Skin-perfecting Tinted Moisturizer SPF 20 (1-954-765-3005; www.shinobayderm.com)

Shino Bay Cosmetic Solutions Antioxidant LightScreen SPF 30 (1-954-765-3005; www.shinobayderm.com)

Avène High Protection Mineral Cream (www.avene.com); through doctors' offices only

Sheer Physical UV Defense SPF 50 (www.skinceutricals.com); through doctors' offices only

Neutrogena Ultra Sheer Dry Touch Sunscreen SPF 100 (www.neutrogena.com)

## PRODUCTS TO TREAT MELASMA AND BROWN DISCOLORATION

N-lighten Me Hydroquinone-free Skin Brightening Lotion (1-954-765-3005; www.shinobayderm.com)

Obagi Nu-Derm systems and Obagi-C Rx systems (www.obagi.com); through doctors' offices only

Triluma (www.triluma.com); through doctors offices only

Cosmelan MD (www.mesoesteticusa.com); through doctors' offices only

Lytera Skin Brightening Complex (www.SkinCeuticals .com); through doctors' offices only

SkinCeuticals Advance Pigment Corrector (www.SkinCeuticals .com); through doctors' offices only

Melanage Skin Brightening System (www.theskincompany.com); through doctors' offices only

### RETINOIDS

Obagi 360 retinol creams (www.obagi.com); through doctors' offices only

Retriderm (www.biopelle.com); through doctors' offices only

SkinMedica Retinol Complex 1.0 (www.skinmedica.com); through doctors' offices only

Neutrogena Rapid Wrinkle Repair (www.neutrogena.com)

Roc Retinol Correction Deep Wrinkle Night Cream (www.rocskincare.com)

Ionzyme C-Quence Skin Care (www.environ.co.za); through doctors' offices only

Retrinal (www.avene usa.com); through doctors' offices only

Retin-A (prescription only); through doctors' offices only

Differin (prescription only); through doctors' offices only

Tazorac (prescription only); through doctors' offices only

### HYDROXY ACIDS

Glytone Skin Care (www.glytone-usa.com); through doctor's offices only

Allergan Vivite (www.viviteskincare.com); through doctor's offices only

Nucelle Mandelic Marine Complex formulations (www.nucelle.com)

Shino Bay Cosmetics Solutions Glycolic Acid Cream and pads (1-954-765-3005; www.shinobayderm.com)

### TCA (TRICHLOROACETIC ACID) CREAMS

Shino Bay Cosmetics Solutions Spotlight Cream and pads (1-954-765-3005; www.shinobayderm.com)

### ANTIOXIDANTS

SkinCeuticals C E Ferulic Serum (www.SkinCeuticals .com); through doctor's offices only

SkinCeuticals Phloterin CF Gel and Serum (www.SkinCeuticals .com); through doctor's offices only

SkinCeuticals Resveratrol B E Serum (www.SkinCeuticals .com); through doctor's offices only

SkinCeuticals C + AHA Serum (www.SkinCeuticals .com); through doctor's offices only

Innovative Skin Care Is Clinical (www.innovativeskincare.com); through doctor's offices only

Glytone C E and Red Tea; through doctor's offices only

### ALPHA LIPOIC ACID

Topical treatments developed by Nicholas Perricone, M.D (www.perriconemd.com, www.sephora.com)

### IDEBENONE

Elizabeth Arden Prevage (www.prevageskin.com)

### GREEN TEA

SkinMedix Replenix CF (www.skinmedix.com); through doctor's offices only

### COFFEEBERRY

Revaleskin Organoceutical (www.revaleskin.com); through doctor's offices only

### NIACINAMIDE

Nia-24 (www.nia24.com); through doctor's offices only

### *PEPTIDES*

Neova Copper Peptide (www.neova.com); through doctor's offices only

Shino Bay Cosmetic Solutions Matrixyl and Dermaxyl (1-954-765-3005; www.shinobayderm.com)

Shino Bay Cosmetic Solutions Make Me Younger (1-954-765-3005; www.shinobayderm.com)

### *MOISTURIZERS FOR SENSITIVE SKIN*

Shino Bay Cosmetic Solutions B-Sensitive moisturizer (1-954-765-3005; www.shinobayderm.com)

Shino Bay Cosmetic Solutions Vitality Soothing Salve (1-954-765-3005; www.shinobayderm.com)

Avène Skin Recovery Cream (www.aveneusa.com); through doctor's offices only

### *MOISTURIZERS FOR ROSACEA AND INTOLERANT SKIN*

Avène Redness Relief Soothing Cream (www.aveneusa.com); through doctor's offices only

# References

---

## CHAPTER 1: FAT IS YOUR FRIEND

A.K. Gosain, M.H. Klein, P.V. Sudhakar, and R.W. Prost. "A Volumetric Analysis of Soft Tissue Changes in the Aging Midface Using High-Resolution MRI: Implications for Facial Rejuvenation," *Plastic and Reconstructive Surgery*, vol. 115 (April 2005): pp. 1143–52.

C. Le Louarn, D. Buthiau, and J. Buis. "Structural Aging: The Facial Recurve Concept," *Aesthetic Plastic Surgery,* vol. 31 (November/December 2007): pp. 213–18.

N.G. Norgan. "The Beneficial Effect of Body Fat and Adipose Tissue in Humans," *International Journal of Obesity*, vol. 21 (1997): pp. 738–46.

J.E. Pessa. "An Algorithm of Facial Aging: Verification of Lambros's Theory by Three-Dimensional Stereolithography, with Reference to the Pathogenesis of Mid Facial Aging, Sclera Show, and Lateral Sub-Orbital through Deformity," *Plastic and Reconstructive Surgery,* vol. 106 (August 2000): pp. 479–88.

D. Vleggaar and R. Fitzgerald. "Facial Volume Restoration of the Aging Face with Poly-L-Lactic Acid," *Dermatologic Therapy,* vol. 24 (January/February 2011): pp. 2–27.

D. Vleggaar. "Soft Tissue Augmentation and the Role of Poly-L-Lactic Acid," *Plastic and Reconstructive Surgery,* vol. 118, supplement (September 2006): pp. 465–545.

K.M. Zelman. "The Skinny on Fat: Good Fats vs. Bad Fats," WebMD.com (accessed February 17, 2014). Website: http://www.webmd.com/diet/features/skinny-fat-good-fats-bad-fats.

## CHAPTER 2: THE "DARN CLOCK"

J.M. Doul, J. Ferri, and M. Laude. "The Influence of Senescence on Craniofacial Aging and Cervical Morphology in Humans," *Surgical and Radiologic Anatomy,* vol. 19 (1997): pp. 175–83.

J.E. Pessa, V.P. Zadoo, C. Yuan, et al. "Concertina Effect and Facial Aging: Non-Linear Aspects of Youthfulness and Skeletal Remodeling, and Why Perhaps Infants Have Jouls," *Plastic and Reconstructive Surgery,* vol. 103 (February 1999): pp. 635–44.

A.J. Pettofrezzo. Vectors and Their Applications (New York: Dover, 2005). H.E. Huntley. *The Divine Proportion: A Study in Mathematical Beauty* (New York: Dover, 1970).

D. Vleggaar and R. Fitzgerald. "Facial Volume Restoration of the Aging Face with Poly-L-Lactic Acid," *Dermatologic Therapy,* vol. 24 (January/February 2011): pp. 2–27.

## CHAPTER 3: ALL ABOUT SKIN

J.L. Bolognia, J.L. Jorizzo, R.P Rapini, et al. (eds.) *Dermatology* (Philadelphia, PA.: Mosby, 2003).

Shakespeare. *Henry V* (c. 1599). One of Shakespeare's historical plays, it focuses on events surrounding the Battle of Agincourt in 1415 during the Hundred Years' War.

*My Big Fat Greek Wedding,* written by Nia Vardalos, directed by Joel Zwick (2002).

## CHAPTER 4: THE SEVEN PLAGUES

J.L. Bolognia, J.L. Jorizzo, R.P. Rapini, et al. (eds.) *Dermatology* (Philadelphia, PA.: Mosby, 2003).

## CHAPTER 5: SOMETHING ABOUT MARY

J.L. Bolognia, J.L. Jorizzo, R.P. Rapini, et al., editors. *Dermatology* (Philadelphia, PA.: Mosby, 2003).

*There's Something about Mary* written by Ed Decter, John J. Strauss, Peter Farrelly, and Robert Farrelly; directed by Peter Farrelly and Robert Farrelly (1998).

Shakespeare, *Antony and Cleopatra.* One of Shakespeare's tragedies, it is based on Plutarch's Lives and focuses on events between the Sicilian Revolt and the suicide of Cleopatra during the Final War of the Roman Republic.

Skin Cancer Foundation. "Shining Light on Ultraviolet Radiation," Skincancer. org (accessed April 2, 2014).

## CHAPTER 6: THROUGH THE YEARS

J. Dover. *The Youth Equation: Take 10 Years Off Your Face* (Hoboken, N.J.: John Wiley & Sons, 2009).

Eric Finzi, M.D., Ph.D., and Erica Wasserman, Ph.D., "Treatment of Depression with Botulinum Toxin A: A Case Series," *Journal of Dermatologic Surgery,* vol. 32, no. 5 (May 2006): pp. 645–50.

## CHAPTER 7: "BOTOX® SAVED MY MARRIAGE"

A. Carruthers and J. Carruthers. *Procedures in Cosmetic Dermatology Series: Botulinum Toxin* (2nd ed.) (Philadelphia, PA.: Elsevier Saunders, 2008).

R. Small and H. Dalano. *A Practical Guide to Botulinum Toxin Procedures* (Philadelphia, PA.: Lippincott Williams and Wilkins, 2012).

L. Baumann. *Cosmetic Dermatology,* second edition. (New York: McGraw-Hill, 2009).

## CHAPTER 8: FILL ME UP

*Death Becomes Her,* written by David Koepp and Martin Donovan; directed by Robert Zemeckis (1992).

## CHAPTER 9: RAYS OF LIGHT

Albert Einstein. "Zur Quantentheorie der Strahlung" ("On the Quantum Theory of Radiation"), *Physikalische Zeitschrift,* vol. 18 (March 3, 1917): pp. 121–8.

J.D. Goldberg. *Procedures in Cosmetic Dermatology Series: Laser and Lights* (Philadelphia, PA.: Elsevier Saunders, 2005).

P.M. Goldman. *Procedures in Cosmetic Dermatology Series: Photodynamic Therapy,* second edition. (Philadelphia, PA.: Saunders Elsevier, 2008).

## CHAPTER 10: LOTIONS AND POTIONS

N. Perricone. *The Wrinkle Cure: Unlock the Power of Cosmeceuticals for Supple, Youthful Skin* (New York: Warner Books, 2001).

Z. Draelos. *Procedures in Cosmetic Dermatology: Cosmeceuticals,* second edition. (Philadelphia, PA.: Saunders Elsevier, 2009).

L. Baumann. *Cosmetic Dermatology,* second edition. (New York: McGraw Hill, 2009).

## CHAPTER 11: BEAUTY IS WHERE YOU FIND IT

L.S. Davis, M. Lubovich. *Hunks, Hotties and Pretty Boys: Twentieth-Century Representations of Male Beauty* (Newcastle upon Tyne, U.K.: Cambridge Scholars Publishing, 2008).

N. Etcoff. *Survival of the Prettiest: The Science of Beauty* (New York: Anchor Books, 2000).

Sam Levenson. *In One Era and Out the Other* (New York: Simon & Schuster, 1973).

Maxwell Maltz, M.D. *Psycho-Cybernetics* (New York: Prentice-Hall, 1960).

D.V.P. Marks. *Human Beauty: An Economic Analysis* [dissertation]. (Cambridge, MA.: Harvard University, 1989).

Yoram Wind and Colin Crook, with Robert Gunther. *The Power of Impossible Thinking: Transform the Business of Your Life and the Life of Your Business* (Upper Saddle River, N.J.: Wharton School Publishing/Pearson Education, 2005).

## CHAPTER 12:COLOR ME PERFECT

G. Hernandez. *Classic Beauty: The History of Make-Up* (Philadelphia, PA.: Schiffer; 2011).

## CHAPTER 13: BE YOUTHFUL

T.A. Baroody, D.C, N.D., Ph.D. *Alkalize or Die: Superior Health Through Proper Alkaline-Acid Balance,* ninth edition (Waynesville, N.C.: Holographic Health, 1991).

A. Hutschnecker. *The Will to Live* (New York: Thomas Y. Crowell Company, 1951).

F.K. Meyer, M.D., "Global Strategy in Preventative Medicine," *Annals of Internal Medicine,* vol. 3, no. 2 (August 1, 1950): pp. 275–91.

C. Vasey, N.D. *The Acid-Alkaline Diet for Optimum Health: Restore Your Health by Creating pH balance in Your Diet*, second edition (Rochester, VT.: Healing Arts Press, 2006).

R. Welch. Raquel: *Beyond the Cleavage* (New York: Weinstein Books, 2010).

# Index

# About the Author

**Shino Bay Aguilera, D.O.,** is a board-certified cosmetic dermatologist and dermatologic surgeon, a fellow of the American Osteopathic College of Dermatology, and an expert in cosmetic laser technology and age-reversal techniques. A former medical director of Nova Southeastern University's dermatology residency program, Dr. Aguilera also has taught dermatology at Lake Erie College of Osteopathic Medicine, the University of Miami, Suncoast University, and the Universidad del Rosario in Colombia. Originally from Panama, he holds a bachelor's degree from the University of California, Los Angeles, and the Western University of Health Sciences.

While attending school, Dr. Aguilera worked as a top fashion and runway model. While pursuing this vocation, he developed a deep understanding of beauty and how to optimize it, and a passion for the art and science of aesthetics. He is a member of the American Academy of Dermatology, the American Osteopathic College of Dermatology, the American Society for Dermatologic Surgery, the American Society of Laser Medicine and Surgery, and the Broward County Dermatology Society.

Dr. Aguilera is founder of the Shino Bay Cosmetic Dermatology, Plastic Surgery & Laser Institute, in Fort Lauderdale, Florida, which has been named a laser center of excellence by Cynosure Lasers, the world's leading laser manufacturer. He is participating in ongoing FDA clinical trial studies whose aim is to determine the best treatment protocols and maximize the safety and efficacy of emerging laser technology. His institute is an advanced physician training center for the United States and Latin America.

A top-requested international physician trainer and keynote speaker, Dr. Aguilera travels the world teaching physicians the proper use of the newest laser advances and cosmetic injectable technologies, such as Sculptra Aesthetic™, Botox®, and Allergan®. He is bilingual and has made frequent appearances on English and Spanish television news programs for networks that include CBS, NBC, MegaTV, and Telemundo. Dr. Aguilera developed two new surgical techniques using fillers, Precise-Sculpt (with Sculptra Aesthetic) and HD Sculpt (with Radiesse™). He is the author or coauthor of numerous articles published in different medical and cosmetic journals.

Dr. Aguilera has received many honors, including the prestigious national award for "Best Nonsurgical Facial Enhancement" from the Aesthetic Academy in 2011 and 2012. He is also a humanitarian. His well-rounded medical expertise includes a multitude of non-profit and volunteer work. Dr. Aguilera has served as an assistant medical director for Hospice of the Palm Beaches and volunteered his services to hurricane shelters helping displaced people. Using his own funds to travel and donating his own supplies, he periodically volunteers skin cancer screenings and other important dermatological services to people in impoverished countries around the world who cannot afford healthcare.

Dr. Aguilera lives and works in greater Miami-Fort Lauderdale, Florida.

**Loren Psaltis** (contributor) spent many years in the beauty industry as a retail buyer for cosmetics, a brand manager for Calvin Klein South Africa, a photographer, a stylist, and a professional makeup artist. She was instrumental in the development of a line of cosmetics for Stuttafords Department Stores in Southern Africa. She has also worked as a sales and motivational training manager and brand development consultant. Currently, she is the marketing director of Cartoon Candy. Loren is the author of *The Devolution Of Man*. She lives in Southern Florida.